Frank Arjava Petter

Reiki
The Legacy of
Dr. Usui

Rediscovered documents on the origins
and developments of the Reiki system,
as well as new aspects of the Reiki energy

Translated by Christine M. Grimm

LOTUS LIGHT
SHANGRI-LA

5th English Printing 2013
4th English Printing 2010
3rd English Printing 2005
2nd English Printing 1999
1st English Edition 1998
© by Lotus Press
Box 325, Twin Lakes, WI 53181 USA
The Shangri-La series is published in cooperation
with Schneelöwe Verlagsberatung, Federal Republic of Germany
© 1998 by Windpferd Verlagsgesellschaft mbH, Aitrang, Germany
All rights reserved
Translated by Christine Grimm
Edited by D. Niemann
Composition and make-up: *panta rhei!* – MediaService Uwe Hiltmann
Cover design by Kuhn Grafik, Digitales Design, Zurich
by using a picture of Tsutomo Oishi

ISBN: 978-0-9149-5556-6
Library of Congress Catalog Number: 98067864

Printed in USA

TABLE OF CONTENTS

Expression of Thanks 7
Preface 9

Chapter 1—Usui Reiki Ryoho Hikkei, Dr. Usui's Handbook
  The Usui Reiki Ryoho Handbook 13
Questions and Answers 14
The Poetry 21

Chapter 2—Reiki History 25
Dr. Usui 26
The Five Reiki Principles 28
The Numerological Character—Analysis of Dr. Usui 31
The Horoscope of Mikao Usui 37
The Traditional Reiki Degrees 38
Authentic or Not Authentic 39

Chapter 3—The Mental Body 45
Sharing 45
Fear 46
Power, Money, and Reiki 49
Reiki Snares 53
Suffering 55
Expressing Feelings 56
The Inner Child 57

Chapter 4—Being Free 61
Conditioning 61
The Power of Thoughts 63
Spiritual Awareness 66
Transience 71

Chapter 5—Experiencing 73
Experiments with Reiki 73
Reiki and Other Living Beings 74
Time to Experience 76
Energy 77
Grounding 79
Feeling Good 81

Chapter 6—Body and Soul   83
Being Healthy and Being Sick   83
Activate the Healing Power of Your Body   88

Chapter 7—My Personal Experiences   93
My Reiki Path   93
Exercises   118
Afterword   123

Expression of Thanks

I would like to express my most sincere gratitude to all of you who have shared your experiences, criticism, and suggestions with me and have supported me with your good wishes and your energy.

A special thank-you goes to my wife Chetna for her love and untiring assistance in times when my Japanese wasn't adequate for the research; to Shizuko Akimoto, who answered the many confusing questions that were nagging me; to T. Oishi for sharing his kind help and generosity and his knowledge and energy with us; to F. Ogawa for the many new bits of information about Dr. Usui; to Walter Lübeck for his advice; to Prem Mangla for drawing up the numerological analysis; to Ginny Bydder for the horoscope; to the Windpferd team for its terrific help in giving the manuscript the finishing touches that led to this book; and to Osho for the spiritual guidance that transformed my confusion into a wonderful adventure. In addition, I would like to thank all my Reiki teachers and friends who initiated me: Lino Alelyunas, Ginny Bydder, Agehanand Popad, William Rand, Engelbert Maugg, and Walter Lübeck. Also to my parents for always supporting me on my spiritual path. And ultimately, I would like to thank Existence, which has been generous time and again in giving me the opportunity of growing toward the light.

In no way do I see the ideas presented in this book as "my own." They have arisen from both the endless conversations with my wife and many other Reiki teachers and the wisdom of many spiritual teachers. It is impossible to personally thank all of these here, so please don't be offended if I haven't mentioned everyone.

Many writers, artists, and musicians share the same outlook when it comes to their art: they feel like a hollow bamboo reed through which the wind plays its song. This is exactly how I how I also see it.

To all of you, dear readers, my most sincere thanks for listening!

Dedicated to my master Osho

Preface

For years I have been asking myself why Reiki is so well-received throughout the entire world. Whether in Europe, North America and South America, or even in Australia and Asia, the Reiki wave is increasing in size and intensity.

There are so many effective forms of therapy, yet Reiki appears to exercise a special impulse. Whatever it may be, Reiki is a method of self-realization, a path to the light, to God, or to oneself. And this is probably the most attractive thing about the Reiki path. Reiki fulfills the longing for non-dogmatic method of further developing ourselves, which is also compatible with our personal philosophy of life or religion.

Reiki requires no background knowledge of philosophy, religion, medicine, or the like, and can be used by any person, of practically any age.

For small children, I personally wouldn't recommend anything beyond the First Reiki degree since keeping the symbols "secret" would probably turn into stress for a child and "revealing" them would create guilt feelings. In addition, according to my experience it's important that a person wants to learn Reiki for himself. The wishes of the parents shouldn't be the decisive factor for the child. In the same way, I wouldn't force a child to go to church or to the temple.

The beautiful thing about Reiki is that we aren't dependent upon a therapist and can treat ourselves. Since the energy flows through us like through a bamboo reed, we don't saddle ourselves with negative energy. We become neither tired nor sick after we have treated someone. A Reiki initiation doesn't open a living being's energy channels but just cleanses and strengthens the naturally existing channels. Reiki works in such a gentle manner that it's almost always well-tolerated.

Working with Reiki is an interesting adventure in any case. The work on ourselves, as well as on others, is fun and constantly gives us insights we hadn't imagined before. Being permitted to work with another person's body is a great honor: in this way, we are allowed to experience the divinity inherent to all of us. Particularly today, living in a society that has become estranged from the physical body, there are some surprises in store for us as we learn to lovingly devote ourselves to our bodies.

For me, the most wonderful thing about Reiki is its many aspects. In my eyes, Reiki isn't identical with healing or the art of healing on the physical and psychological level. It not only effects the physical body but also goes beyond it to the emotional and mental areas, and even much further than that. Healing is just a small, but important aspect of the Reiki work in the interaction of healing and disease. Especially with the help of the Second Degree, we learn to direct energies to many levels.

Healing, energy work, body work, therapy, and so forth are just the attributes in which we clothe Reiki so that it's easier to understand and be comprehended by the rational mind.

An artist will learn to more effectively transform energy into art, a businessperson will turn Reiki into money, and a cook will create energetically charged dishes. A master of the art of living will turn Reiki into enjoyment of life!

As I see it, the Reiki path is the path of becoming a human being. Although we already come to the Earth as human beings, this state of being human is just the potential. We are permitted to strive for its realization in this life.

By means of the Reiki power, we have the possibility of uniting heaven and earth. The Tree of Life sends its roots deep into the Earth. Without the Earth, the energy of development, there would be no evolution for us human beings. Reiki is our energetic root here on Earth, and the deeper we are rooted in the Earth, the higher we can let our crown stretch into the sky.

The theoretical roots of Reiki are found in a colorful mixture of Mikkyo Buddhism, Chinese Qigong, and Japanese Shintoism.

However, I would like to leave the introduction to this book up to the founder of Usui Reiki Ryoho, Mikao Usui. After years of searching, we finally found a manuscript with the title of Reiki Ryoho Hikkei in July of 1997. This manuscript was written about seventy-five years ago by the Usui Sensei (teacher, master), as he was called by his students. This handbook was handed out to all of his students at that time.

I would like to expressly emphasize at this point that this is not channeled material.

During the course of this book, I use the name of Dr. Usui for Usui Sensei, although he wasn't a physician in the current sense of the word. However, in my opinion, he was a doctor in the best way possible: He sacrificed himself with all his strength to the task of healing his fellow human beings on all levels—in body, mind, and soul. I find it inappropriate to use his Japanese title as a form of address outside of Japan.

The Reiki Ryoho Handbook consists of three sections: The first part is an explanation to the public, which shall serve as an introduction here. The second part contains questions and answers and is reproduced here in the second chapter. The third part consists of spiritual Japanese poetry, called waka, and you will find some of these selected poems in the third chapter.

My parents-in-law, Kaneo and Masano Kobayashi, as well as my wife Chetna and I, provided the translation of this manuscript from the Japanese. I have put my comments in parentheses.

It's hard for me to believe that we should be the first people from the West to have this manuscript fall into their hands. Yet, however that may be, I am very happy that we have finally succeeded in finding something written by Dr. Usui's hand since the current developments demand this. In an age in which the world-wide protection of (claim to) the "brandname" of "Reiki" is being aimed for and by a certain group, I would like to stimulate your thoughts, dear reader, with this introduction. As Dr. Usui personally sais in his introduction, Reiki can never and will never belong to just one person or one organization. Reiki is the spiritual heritage of all of humanity. But we will now let Dr. Usui speak for himself...

Chapter 1

Reiki Ryoho Hikkei*, Dr. Usui's Handbook (The Reiki Ryoho Handbook)

Why I teach this method (Reiki) publicly; explanation by the founder Usui Mikao.
From time immemorial, it has often happened that someone who has found an original, secret law has either kept it for himself or only shared it with his descendents.

This secret was then used as security in life for his descendents. (Descendents means not only one's own family but also one's own students here. The phrase "security in life" is meant in the sense of securing one's own financial future.) The secret is not passed on to outsiders. However, this is an old-fashioned custom from the last century (and therefore outdated).

In times like these, the happiness of humanity is based on working together and the desire for social progress.

This is why I would never allow anyone to possess it (Reiki) just for himself!

Our Reiki Ryoho is something absolutely original and cannot be compared with any other (spiritual) path in the world.

This is why I would like to make this method (freely) available to the public for the well-being of humanity. Each of us has the potential of being given a gift by the divine, which results in the body and soul becoming unified. In this way (with Reiki), a great many people will experience the blessing of the divine.

First of all, our Reiki Ryoho is an original therapy, which is built upon the spiritual power of the universe.

Through it, the human being will first be made healthy, and then peace of mind and joy in life will be increased.

Today we need improvements and restructuring in our lives so that we can free our fellow human beings from illness and emotional suffering.

This is the reason why I dare to freely teach this method in public.

---

* The Japanese word hikkei means handbook.

Questions and Answers

The following questions about Reiki have been answered by Dr. Usui himself. The exact date and the name of the interviewer were not mentioned. According to the date mentioned in the text (see page 17) we know that it must have been between 1922 and Dr. Usui's death in 1926. Since the original text is about 75 years old and written in Old Japanese, we have had to make some minor changes so that the text is easier to understand. My notes have been put into parentheses. Chetna and I did the translation into English.

Question: What is Usui Reiki Ryoho?
Answer: With thankfulness we receive and live according to principles (the Reiki Principles, see chapter 2) prescribed by the Meiji Emperor.

In order to achieve the proper (spiritual) path for humanity, we must live according to these principles. This means that we must learn to improve our spirit* and body with practice. To do this, we first heal the spirit.

Afterwards, we make the body healthy. When our mind finds itself on the healthy path of honesty and seriousness, the body will become healthy completely on its own. So the mind and body are one, and we live out our life in peace and joy. We heal ourselves and the illnesses of others, intensifying and increasing our own happiness in life, as well as that of others. This is the goal of the Usui Reiki Ryoho.

---

* The Japanese word kokoro is used here. In many translations from Japanese, this is often wrongly translated with "heart." However, this is just half of the truth. In Western cultures we divide the human spirit into two parts—heart and head, emotions and thoughts. The Japanese person doesn't make this differentiation and considers heart and head to be a unity merged with each other.

This unity is called kokoro. I wish that my emotions and thoughts would always be integrated and at one! This completely different way of experiencing the world and oneself has very far-reaching consequences: if, for example, we ask a Japanese person what he thinks or feels, we often will not get a clear response because the boundaries between feelings and thoughts are not clearly defined. I will go into the topic of cultural differences in the chapter "Authentic or Not Authentic."

Question: Is Usui Reiki Ryoho the same as hypnotherapy, kiai jutsu, (concentrating "Ki" in the abdomen and letting out a yell) or shinko ryoho (religious therapy) and so forth? Is it a similar form of therapy under a different name?

Answer: No, no. It is not similar to the forms of therapy described above.

At the end of many years of hard training, I found a spiritual secret:

This (Reiki) is a method of freeing the body and mind*.

Question: Is it (Reiki) a shinrei ryoho (a psychic, spiritual method of healing?)

Answer: Correct, we could call it shinrei ryoho. However, it would also be possible to call it physical therapy since energy and light radiate from all the body parts of the person who is giving the treatment.

Energy and light mainly radiate from the eyes, the mouth, and the hands of the giver of the treatment. At the same time, the treatment-giver either fixes his eyes for two or three minutes on the afflicted parts of the body, blows on them, or gently massages them.

Toothaches, headaches, stomachaches, swelling of the chest, nerve pain, bruises, cuts, burns, and so forth, simply heal.

However, chronic diseases are not as easy to treat. But the fact is that even one single treatment of a chronic disease shows a (positive) effect.

I ask myself how this phenomenon can be explained in the sense of medical science. Well, the reality is always more impressive than fiction could ever be. If you would see the results (that a Reiki treatment brings), you would have to agree with me. Even someone who does not want to believe it cannot deny the reality (the result, the truth).

Question: Is it necessary to believe in Usui Reiki Ryoho so that healing can occur?

Answer: No, since it (Usui Reiki Ryoho) is different than other psychic methods of healing, psychotherapy, and hypnotherapy.

---

* In the Japanese text, the term rei as in Reiki is used here.

Assent and faith are not necessary since it (Reiki) does not work with suggestions. It makes no difference whether a person is antagonistic and mistrustful or refuses to believe in it. For example, it functions just as well with small children or people who are seriously ill and unconscious.

Of ten people, perhaps one person will bring trust (in the success of the healing) along with him to the first treatment. Even after their first treatment, most people will already feel the (positive) effect and the trust within them grows (on its own).

Question: Which health disorders can be healed with the help of Usui Reiki Ryoho?
Answer: All diseases, whether they have been caused by psychological or physical factors, can be healed with the Usui Reiki Ryoho.

Question: Does Usui Reiki Ryoho only heal diseases?
Answer: No, it not only heals diseases of the physical body. It can also heal bad habits and psychological disorders like despair, weakness (in the sense of weakness of character), cowardice, difficulty in making decisions, and nervousness.

With this (with Reiki energy), the spirit (kokoro) becomes similar to God or Buddha and we develop the goal in life of healing our fellow human beings. This (through the Buddha similarity) is how we make ourselves and others happy.

Question: How does the Usui Reiki Ryoho heal?
Answer: I was not initiated into this method by anyone in the universe. I also did not have to make any efforts to achieve supernormal healing powers (siddhis). While I fasted, I touched an intense energy and in a mysterious manner, I was inspired (I received the Reiki energy). As in a coincidence, it became clear to me that I had been given the spiritual art of healing. Although I am the founder of this method, I find it hard to explain all of this more precisely. Physicians and scholars research (in this field) passionately, but it has been difficult (up to now) to come to a conclusion that is based on medical science. The time will come when it (Reiki) will meet with science.

Question: Does the Usui Reiki Ryoho use medications? And are there any kind of side effects?
Answer: It uses neither medications nor instruments. It uses only looking, blowing, stroking, (light) tapping, and touching (of the afflicted parts of the body). This is what heals diseases.

Question: Does a person need medical knowledge in order to use the Usui Reiki Ryoho?
Answer: Our ryoho (healing method) is a spiritual method that goes beyond medical science. It therefore is not based upon it.

When you either look at, blow on, touch, or stroke the afflicted part of the body, you will achieve the desired goal. For example, you touch the head when you want to treat the brain, the abdomen when you want to treat the abdomen, and the eyes for the eyes. You take neither bitter medicine nor use hot moxibustion*, and you will be healthy again within a short time. This is why this reiho (spiritual method) is our original creation.

Question: How do renowned physicians see it (the Usui Reiki Ryoho)?
Answer: The educated authorities in this field appear (in the evaluation of the Usui Reiki Ryoho) to be very fair. (These days) well-known European physicians are very critical toward the (stubborn) prescription of medications. As an aside, Dr. Sen Nagai from the Medical Teikoku University said: "We physicians know how to diagnose an illness, record it empirically and understand it, but we do not know how to treat it."

(Another physician) Dr. Kondo said: "It is very arrogant to say that medicine has made tremendous progress since modern medicine neglects the spiritual equilibrium (of the patient). This is its greatest disadvantage." Doctor Sakae Hara said: "It is an impertinence to treat a human being, who possesses spir-

---

* Moxibustion, a healing art that is employed in Tibet, China, and Japan, makes use of a philosophy and technique similar to acupuncture. However, no fine needles are inserted into the body here but a tiny amount of mogusa (moxa herb, a type of wormwood) is burnt on certain meridians and acupuncture points in a specific sequence and frequency.

itual wisdom, like an animal. I believe that we can reckon with a great revolution in the field of therapy in the future."

Dr. Rokura Kuga said: "It is a fact that non-physicians (therapists) have carried out a series of therapies such as psychotherapy with a high degree of success that has not even been achieved by medical faculties because these therapies include the character, the personal symptoms of the patient, and many different (healing) methods in their treatment.

If they (as physicians associated with the medical faculty) would blindly reject therapists and psychotherapists (who are not associated) and attempt to impede them in their work, this would be very narrow-minded."*

Physicians and pharmacists often understand this and come to be initiated (by me, by us into Reiki).

Question: What does the government think about it (the Usui Reiki Ryoho)?
Answer: On the sixth of February in the eleventh year of the Taisho period (1922), the representative Teiji Matsushita posed the following question to the meeting of the Federal Parliament about the budget: "What is the position of the government on therapists who currently practice psychotherapy and spiritual therapy (like that of the Usui Reiki Ryoho) without a (physician's) license?

Mr. Ushio of the government committee answered as follows: "Hypnotherapy and the like (similar therapy forms) were judged to be bad forms of therapy more than ten years ago, but today they have been better researched, and also effectively applied in psychiatry. It is difficult to want to solve everything related to the human being with medications. Physicians follow certain paths, which are based on medical principles, in order to heal disease. The use of touch and electrotherapy in combatting disease are not components of the healing methods of the medical faculty."

This is why the Usui Reiki Ryoho is subject to neither the laws applying to the medical faculty nor to those regarding acupuncture and moxibustion.

---

* Nihon Iji Shinpo (a medical journal with the title of "Japanese Medical News")

Question: In this type of therapy, the spiritual healing abilities are certain to just come to those people who have been spiritually developed from the time of their birth. I do not believe that someone can learn this. Or do you think so?
Answer: No, no.*

All beings into whom life has been breathed have received as a gift the spiritual ability to heal. The same applies to plants, animals, fish, and insects.

But human beings, who represent the culmination point of Creation, have the greatest power. The Usui Reiki Ryoho appeared in the world in order to make this (the power given to human beings on their path) useful.

Question: Can anyone be initiated into Usui Reiki Ryoho?
Answer: Naturally. Men and women, old and young, physicians and uneducated people who live according to the moral principles can certainly learn within a short time to heal themselves, as well as others. To date, I have initiated one thousand and several hundred of people, and not one individual failed to experience the desired result. Anyone, even someone who has just learned Shoden (the First Degree) has apparently received the ability of healing diseases. If we think about it, it is quite strange that we can learn to heal illness within such a short time, although this is the most difficult thing (in the world) for human beings. Even I find this astonishing. This is the characteristic thing about our spiritual healing method, that we can learn something so difficult in such a simple way.

Question: With it (the Usui Reiki Ryoho), other people can be healed. But what about oneself? Can a person also heal his own health disorders?
Answer: If we cannot heal our own diseases, then how should we heal others?

---

*In Japanese, a question that someone wants to answer with "yes" is sometimes answered with "no." This is a linguistic subtlety of the language.

Question: What must be done in order to learn (the Second Degree) Okuden?
Answer: Okuden consists of a number of (healing) methods: Hatsuleiho, (light) tapping, stroking, pressing with the hands, distance healing, the healing of habits (mental healing), and so forth. First learn Shoden and when you bring (to me, the teacher) good results, behave properly, honestly and morally, and are enthusiastic (about Reiki), then you will be initiated (by me, by us into Okuden).

Question: Is there even more (to learn) in the Reiki Ryoho than Okuden?
Answer: There is (still) Shinpiden (the highest degree).

The interview ends here.

The Poetry

The handbook of the Usui Reiki Ryoho includes 125 poems in the Japanese waka form. The waka is a somewhat longer poem than the haiku, with which we are more familiar in the West and which must always consist of 5 syllables in the first, 7 syllables in the second, and 5 syllables in the third line. The waka has 5-7-5-7-7 syllables. Both poetry forms frequently have spiritual themes and are composed with the help of certain words (see waka no 2).

You may ask what these poems have to do with Reiki, but since Dr. Usui gave them to his students, I don't want to keep them from you. These poems were composed by the Meiji Emperor, who wanted to give his people instructions for a life worthy of a human being. My wife Chetna and her parents selected the first 14 poems of these in order to give us a good overview of the existing material. Since the actual style cannot be reproduced in English, I have again included the transcribed version. In addition, by this means I would like to avoid any possible doubt about the authenticity of this text from the beginning.

Each waka has been given a number and a title in the sense of interrelated subjects. The translation from the Old Japanese was done by Kaneo and Masano Kobayashi, and Chetna and I did the translation into English. Since I am an enthusiastic poet, when it appeared to be the right thing to do, I changed the length of the five lines in order to make the text more clear. Japanese grammar cannot be compared at all with that of the Indo-European languages. Texts like the following can certainly be interpreted, understood, and translated in a variety of ways. Since I always am very amused at the meanings that critics read into my own poetry, I have added no further commentary. The meaning of each poem is, and should be, different for each of us. So we should each experience it in our own personal way.

(My comments are in parentheses.)

1 Tsuki

Akinoyono
Tsuki wa mukashi ni
Kawaranedo
Yo ni naki hito no
Ooku narinuru

2 Ten

Asamidori
Sumiwataritaru
Oozola no
Hiroķi onoga
Kokoro tomogana

3 Worini furete

Atsushitomo
Iware zari keri
Nie kaeru
Mizuta ni tateru
Shizu wo omoeba

4 Ochiba Kaze

Amatatabi
Shigurete someshi
Momijiba wo
Tada hitokaze no
Chirashi kerukana

5 Wori ni furete

Amadari ni
Kubomeri ishi wo
Mitemo shire
Kataki waza tote
Omoi sutemeya

1 The Moon

Profound change occurs
Because so many people
Have gone from this world
But the moon in an autumn night
Remains (always) the same

2 The Sky

Light-green and cloudless
The big sky
I too would like to have
Such a spirit (kokoro)

3 In General

Whenever I think
Of the suffering farmers
In the rice paddies
I cannot say it is hot
Even if this is the case

4 The Wind of Falling Leaves

It takes so much rain
To give the perfect color
To the maple leaves
But they are blown away
By a single gust of wind

5 In General

Understand (life) by
Seeing how the stone has been
Hollowed out by rain
Do not cling to the illusion
That nothing changes

6 Wori ni furete

Ten wo urami
Hito wo togamuru
Koto mo araji
Waga ayamachi wo
Omoi kaeseba

6 In General

I do not need
To be angry at the heavens
Or put the blame on
Others (for my suffering)
If I see my own faults

7 Wori ni Furete

Ayamatamu
Koto mo koso are
Yononaka wa
Amari ni mono wo
Omai sugusaba.

7 In General

There is so much
Blame in this world
So do not worry
About it too much

8 Tomo

Ayamachi wo
Isame kawashite
Shitashimu ga
Makoto no tomo no
Kokoro naruramu

8 Friendship

Being friends
Being able to show
Each other our errors
Is the true shrine
Of friendship

9 Ganjyo matsu/iwawo no ue no matsu

Arashi fuku
Yo nimo ugokuna
Hito gokoro
Iwawo ni nezasu
Matsu no gotoku-ni

9 A Pine Tree on a Rock

Stormy world
Human mind (kokoro)
Remain as still
As the pine tree
Rooted on a rock

10 Nami

Aruruka to
Mireba nagiyuku
Unabara no
Nami koso hito no
Yo ni nitarikere

10 The Wave

One moment stormy
The next moment it is calm
The wave in the ocean
Is actually
Just like human existence

11 Wori no furete

Ie tomite
Akanu kotonaki
Minari tomo
Hito no tsutome ni
Okotaru na yume

11 In General

If the background
You come from is wealthy
And without personal problems
Your human obligations
Are easily forgotten

12 Kyodai

Ie no kaze
Fukisohamu yo mo
Miyuru kana
Tsuranaru eda no
Shigeru ai tsutsu

12 Siblings

Sometimes in this world
The wind shakes the house
But troubles are overcome
If the branches (siblings) of
the tree (family)
Grow up harmoniously

13 Kokoro

Ikanaramu
Koto aru toki mo
Utsusemi no
Hito no kokoro yo
Yutaka naranamu

13 The Spirit (Kokoro)

Whatever happens
In any situation
It is my wish that
(In all its dimensions)
The spirit (kokoro) remains
Without boundaries (free)

14 Kusuri

Iku kusuri
Motomemu yori mo
Tsune ni mi no
Yashinai kusa wo
Tsumeyo tozo omou

14 Medicine

Instead of buying
A great deal of medicine
It is better to take care
Of your (own) body

Chapter 2

REIKI HISTORY

The Reiki Family Tree of the Usui Reiki Ryoho Gakkai

Mikao Usui

Mr. Ushida

Mr. Taketomi

Mr. Watanabe

Mr. Wanami

Ms. Kojama

Mr. Kondo

Teachers of the Usui Reiki Ryoho Gakkai who had their own students:

Mr. Imaizumi, Mr. and Mrs. Isoda, Mr. Shiki, Mr. Kaneko, Ms. Morisako, Mr. Chujiro Hayashi*, Mr. K. Ogawa**, Mr. Tsuboi

Further teachers were/are: Mr. Eguchi, Mr. Hanai, Mr. Harada, Mr. Haraguchi, Mr. Hida, Mr. Ichinose, Mr. Ichiraizaki, Mr. Isobe, Mr. Jo, Mr. Kobayashi, Mr.Kosone, Mr. Matsuo, Ms. Nagano, Ms. Nagamine, Ms. Nakagawa, Mr. Nomura, Mr. F. Ogawa, Mr. Onizuka, Mr. Senju, Mr. Takayama, Ms. Tamura, Ms. Uchida, Mr. Usui and Mr. Yoshizaki.

And here are the official successors to Mikao Usui who have been the presidents of the Usui Reiki Ryoho. The seventh president, who is therefore the rightful successor of Mikao Usui, Mr. Kondo, has been in office since the beginning of 1998.

Dr. Usui

For many of us, the person of Dr. Usui is still that of a fabled creature shrouded in mystic fog. However, he was first of all a human being like you and me! Unfortunately, we still know very little about his life.

We know that he was born on August 15, 1865 in the Japanese province of Gifu, married Sadako Suzuki, and had two children. On March 9, 1926, he died in Fukuyama as a result of cerebral apoplexy. Exactly when Dr. Usui began to teach Reiki is still unclear. We assume that it must have been around the year 1920, which means relatively shortly before his death. In 1921, he opened a Reiki practice in Harajuku, Tokyo, close to the beautiful Meiji Jingu (Meiji shrine). His renown swept through the country like a whirlwind, and he moved to a larger house in Nakano in 1925.

---

* Not only the entire Western Reiki line can be followed back to Mr. Hayashi, but also the Australian line, which is called Enersence. This line developed through Hayashi-Takeuchi-Takamori-Premaratna. A further student of Mr. Hayashi was a Mr. Tatsumi.
** Our contacts in Shizuoka, Mr. F. Ogawa and Mr. T. Oishi learned from Mr. K. Ogawa.

It is written on the Usui memorial stone at the Saihoji Cemetery in Tokyo that his son took over the family business. However, this was not concerned with Reiki. We still haven't been able to find out what type of business he had, but our research continues. I have the feeling that it's time for the secrecy surrounding Dr. Usui to be aired. From all corners of the Reiki world, more and more information has come to light, and the last word has certainly not yet been spoken.

Here in Japan, much of what we had heard about Dr. Usui has turned out to be false or incomplete in the meantime. For example, Dr. Usui wasn't a Christian and he didn't teach at the Doshisha University in Kyoto. He also wasn't registered as a student there. The University of Chicago (where he supposedly studied) knows just as little about him.

The false information came not only from outside Japan. "A reliable source" also assured me that Dr. Usui's first name was pronounced Mikaomi and not Mikao. Theoretically, both are possible since the Chinese kanji often permit more than one pronunciation. However, it proved to be wrong in this case.

The head of the Shizuoka branch of the organization founded by Dr. Usui, Fumio Ogawa, to whom we owe our deepest thanks for his information about Dr. Usui, also told us about a portion of Dr. Usui's life that we hadn't heard of before. He said that for a while Mikao Usui had been the private secretary of the politician Shimpei Goto, who was the Secretary of the Railroad, the Postmaster General, and the Secretary of the Interior and State. In the year Taisho 9 (1922), Mr. Goto became the mayor of Tokyo. We can also assume that Dr. Usui had good relations with many influential politicians and perhaps his travels outside of Japan, which he presumably embarked on according to the inscription on his tombstone, can be explained this way. However, we still do not know exactly what his duties were in the service of Mr. Goto.

The Five Reiki Principles

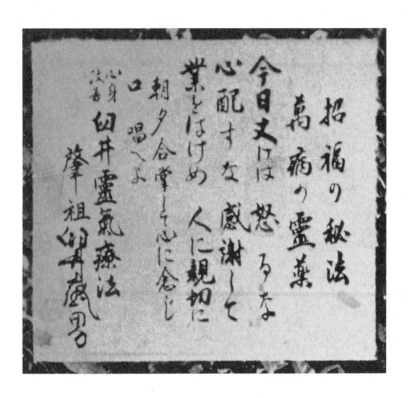

At this point, I would like to once again refer to the five Reiki principles in Usui's handwriting. Because I am so frequently asked about them, I would like to present them here in readable Japanese and in the English language. My notes are in parentheses.

Shoufuku no hihoo	The secret method of inviting happiness
Manbyo no ley-yaku	*The wonderful medicine for all diseases (of the body and the soul)*
Kyo dake wa	*Just today*
1 Okoru-na	*1 Don't get angry*
2 Shimpai suna	*2 Don't worry*
3 Kansha shite	*3 Show appreciation*
4 Goo hage me	*4 Work hard (on yourself)*
5 Hito ni shinsetsu ni	*5 Be kind to others*
Asa yuu gassho shite, koko-ro ni nenji, kuchi ni tonaeyo.	*Mornings and evenings, sit in the gassho position*** and repeat these words out loud and in your heart.*
Shin shin kaizen, Usui Reiki* Ryoho	*(For the) improvement of body and soul, Usui Reiki Ryoho.*
Chosso **Usui Mikao	*The founder, Mikao Usui.*

---

*The Japanese word Reiki can have several different meanings. It consists of two kanji: rei and ki. Rei can mean either spirit, soul, or ghost. Ki can mean energy, atmosphere, mind, heart, soul, feeling, or mood. The word Ryoho means either method, treatment, or system in the sense of a healing system.
** The family name is normally mentioned first in Japanese.
***The Japanese gassho position should be understood as follows: It's best to either sit on the floor with crossed legs or on your legs without crossing them. Now fold your hands in front of your heart chakra. You can naturally also sit on a chair or stand up. As always, the most important thing here is the mental attitude.

As we have already heard from Dr. Usui, a healthy body is followed by a healthy mind. One reason why he probably took over the Meiji Emperor's five rules for life is, in my opinion, that he wanted to give the members of his organization a solid ethical foundation. I believe that Reiki has been preserved for us because of this reason and hasn't, like many other methods of healing, been buried along with its founder. He certainly didn't intend to control his students with the Reiki principles. And I don't think he wanted to found a new religion. Japanese emperors have traditionally been seen as Shinto deities. The Meiji Emperor, for example, was actually said to have been a definite clairvoyant and wonderful healer. The English missionary Dr. John Bachelor, who worked for many years on Hokkaido (where my wife and I live) with the Ainu* is said to have automatically received a Rei-Ju (=initiation) when he was presented a medal by the emperor.

After this initiation, he began to spontaneously heal Ainu and other people seeking help, without ever having received formal training for this purpose.

As with a mantra or a Second Degree Reiki symbol, with the Reiki principles the mind is directed to a specific, meditative basic attitude that is meant to prepare the ground for healing and health on an etheric level. Once the meditative stone begins to roll, the further work can take place. The path always initially goes into the spiritual heart, which should be understood as something like a substation. The rawer energies from the lower chakras are tuned to a higher frequency here. In any situation in life, it is helpful to let ourselves be guided by our heart. In the heart, as the spiritual center of the human being, there is no place for duality; there are no power and money struggles, there is no hatred, no greed, and no other ego-centered difficulties. Whenever a question arises about a portion of life's path, you can become immersed in your heart by repeating the Reiki principles.

If you are no fan of principles, then use the Second Reiki Degree to connect yourself with your heart and imagine that you are breathing the mental-healing symbol into your heart

---

* The Ainu are the original inhabitants of the Japanese chain of islands; there is almost nothing known about the origin of this tribe. Their culture is very similar to that of Native Americans. They live mainly on Hokkaido now.

chakra. There your blood will be enriched with love and harmony, supplying your entire body. Take a few minutes time to feel how love and harmony flow through you in a nourishing way.

Our greatest problem is probably forgetfulness. When we find ourselves in our heart, it isn't possible to have unharmonious thoughts and do bad things to other people. The one quality excludes the other, and with the ability to move ourselves into our heart, we grow beyond the laziness of the human robot. If we could just think of this more often!

Another possibility of moving into your heart is to surround yourself with things that support your heart. Among these things may be pictures or photos of enlightened people or those you love, flowers, plants, gemstones, certain music, or simply the influence of nature.

The Numerological Character Analysis of Dr. Usui

When a Reiki-teacher friend, Engelbert Maugg, recently asked me the meaning of the name "Usui," I could only answer him with a silly remark: Usui could possibly mean "thin." So I then asked Chetna about the meaning of the Chinese characters Mikao and Usui. One of the difficulties with Japanese is the fact that a Chinese character (kanji) can have an entire variety of meanings and ways of writing it. This means that the pronunciation and way of writing it can have a number of meanings. Words are often composed of a number of characters. Usui, for example, consists of "usu" and "i". The "i" in Usui could theoretically mean either the rational mind, wanting, meaning, doctor, medicine, bile, gallbladder, stomach, majesty, rank, reed, or fountain. In this case, the "i" means "well". "Usu" means pestle, in this case a wooden pestle that is used to make rice cake (mochi).

The first name "Mika" is identical with the character "kame" and means vase or vessel. Here this means a ceramic vessel in which water was stored in earlier times. The "o" stands for "man."

In his first name we then recognize a man in which something vital to life and preserving of life—namely water—is stored. His last name tells of the integration of water and rice, body and soul.

After analyzing his name, I suddenly became interested in this process. It occurred to me to ask a dear friend, Ma Prem Mangla, to illuminate the names of Dr. Usui in terms of numerology.

In brief, numerology is a method that has two different origins and systems. The one lies in the Kabbalah, and this method is not very prevalent today. The other is ascribed to the Greek mathematician and forefather of Western mysticism, Pythagoras. On the whole, this system involves assigning a number to every letter of the Latin alphabet, which has a certain meaning and bears a specific energy within itself. This means the number one is associated with "A," the number two with the "B," and so forth. If, for example, we then add the numbers of all the letters in a name, we get a figure that indicates a person's path in life. A difference is also made between consonants and vowels in order to receive various information. This system offers an experienced numerologist a map of the psychological, psychic, and spiritual person, and this map is unbelievably accurate.

Here is the analysis:

The birth name: *Mikao Usui*
The date of birth: *August 15, 1865*
The date of death: *March 9, 1926*
The path in life: *25/7*

Dr. Usui's main learning process in this life, the main reason why he was born in his body, consisted of finding the inner wisdom and the inner understanding that can only be achieved when a person follows his own light and trusts in his own life experience. This path is the path of wisdom, of being alone, and of meditation. It is basically the path of the spiritual seeker, of someone who is open to learning from life instead of collecting knowledge second hand. It is the type of learning that understands that wisdom and true knowledge can only be comprehended when the body, mind, and heart are in harmonious unity with each other.

His special path of learning lead through the ability of being open and receptive (2) in the present moment (5). And Reiki can actually be seen as this as well: understanding and wisdom, coupled with the ability of channeling the energy present in this moment.

The number 7 has the qualities of the esoteric, as well as the tendency toward accuracy. Based on this aspect of his character, this is where the detailed symbolism and the precise systematics, which are a component of Reiki, originated. The teaching of experienced knowledge also plays a role here.

But this energy involves not only the role of teacher, but rather a highly developed person who is capable of passing on his personal light and knowledge to his fellow human beings.

The first pinnacle of his life
(The number 5 with the number 2 as a challenge):

He spent the first 29 years of his life in the energy of the number 5, which describes the exploration of the life energy in a very subtle and sensitive manner. The energy of the number 5 teaches us how to be completely in the present moment and react spontaneously, which is only possible when we are connected and familiar with the energy of our body at every moment. The number 2 as a challenge says that he was unusually receptive and sensitive. The result of this receptivity was that it was possible for him to research life energy on such a fine level that it opened up to him the presence of the subtle flow of energy. This fine and delicate sensing of the life force or life energy was therefore the fundamental experience of his youth. It was natural for him during this time to become familiar with the concept of the life energy flowing through him and connecting it with the energy surrounding him.

The second pinnacle of his life
(the number 8 with the number 4 as a challenge):

During the nine years from his thirtieth to his thirty-eight year of life, he learned what it means to find and live his personal power. In this time period, he probably had to face certain confrontations on the practical and worldly level. He probably became aware of his own direction in life and his own objectives, as well as the possibilities for translating these into action. It is probable that he already began at this time to deal with his fellow human beings from the standpoint of his own inner power and overcome his inherent shyness and secrecy. In order to find this strength within himself, he was forced to live more and more in his physical body, becoming aware of both his inner and his outer reality. He was probably torn away more and more from rigid spiritual concepts in order to increasingly follow his own experiences and his own feelings.

This was a time for him in which he became rooted with the earth, learned to rely upon himself, and become secure within himself and with the way in which he experienced reality and the strength that it brings with it.

The third pinnacle of his life
(the number 4 with the number 2 as a challenge):

The nine years from 39 to 47 were a time of maturity and trust in his subtle, inner reality.

The energy of the number 4 helped him in a free and unconstrained way to live in the natural physical reality, and the challenge of the number 2 helped him in that this took place in an increasingly accentuated sensitive manner. It was during this time that he increasingly came into contact with his deep inner longing (the longing of the soul—number 4) to find his task in life and the reason for his existence. It is also probable that during this phase his true talent, the ability of channeling life energy (expression of the number 11/2) developed and matured. The sensitivity to the life energy had been given to him since childhood, but the ability to consciously let this energy flow through the body and impart it in this way was a process based on the constant sound trust in himself and the experiences he had.

The fourth pinnacle in life
(the number 1 with the number 6 as a challenge):

Starting in his 48th year of life, Dr. Usui began to more intensely develop his own individuality. He mainly lived in his "yang" energy. After the maturation and solidification of the trust in his own life experience of the previous nine years, he was now ready to share his work with his fellow human beings, to tell the world who he is and set his Reiki movement in motion.

The essence of the 1's energy is the self-confidence that we acquired when we have found ourselves and the leadership qualities that result from this. Combined with the number 7 of his personality and his path in life, he became an increasingly independent individual. He may even have been somewhat eccentric.

This energy is also related to initiation. It probably is no coincidence that he not only initiated an entire movement but also initiated individuals into his personal discovery. This only became possible for him in that he integrated the energy of the number 6 (challenge), the energy of the heart, and the necessity of assuming full responsibility for his deeds and inner truth.

The love of his fellow human beings and life itself must have been a very distinct quality of his individuality before the Existence allowed him to find his own direction.

Although he was always very open and sensitive toward others, and was possibly overly sensitive in this respect during his youth, he was probably uncompromising in his later years when approaching the truth of his heart. As we can read in the handbook printed at the beginning of this book, he was probably very clear and precise in understanding the truth of his work and have carried it out and also passed it on in this same way.

Maturity (9)

The number 9 (maturity) says that from the end of his Thirties Dr. Usui was increasingly interested in the physical and emotional condition of his fellow human beings and the state of the world. The 9 is the number of sympathy, of caring and helping on the larger level. Just healing wouldn't have satisfied him: the energy of the 9 would have stimulated him to propagate his knowledge on the larger level by sharing it with others.

His natural intuitive grasp and sympathy for others and their path in life probably also grew in this way.

The life expression (11/2)

Dr. Usui's energy in relation to the work, or the gift that he was permitted to give the world, was the ability to channel higher energy. The energy of 11/2 is the ability to be like a hollow bamboo reed and channel higher energy in either an energetic or intuitive manner through the physical body. Every individual with this life expression (11/2) has this potential; whether it develops or not depends on the rest of the data. The 11/2 is a so-called master number, a high developmental level of yin or feminine energy. This means being firmly rooted with the Earth and the feeling of one's own self (the doubled 1) that the sensitivity and sensitiveness of the 2 energy made it possible for him to tap into the higher dimensions or the divine in the vertical direction instead of letting his energy flow horizontally in the direction of human beings and the Earth.

Starting in his 48th year of life, this ability became increasingly pronounced. He was actually a born channeler who was capable of transforming these experiences by means of the depths of his meditation and perceptive faculty.

The longing of the soul (31/4):
The longing of the soul describes the deep yearning for seeing the truth, experiencing it, and being connected with the degree of reality that can most simply be understood with the help of the religions (Shintoism and Buddhism) surrounding him. This reality is concealed behind the complexity of the rational mind: the simple existence of all things. Up to the point in which this simple existence is lived and experienced, the human being attempts to find his task in life and his lifework. Accordingly, Dr. Usui would have also have seriously sought after his task in life and the meaning of his life. This search probably had its culmination during the third life pinnacle (39-47), the time in which he developed and established his work.

The personality (7)
Since the number 7 is the number of his path in life, as well as the number of his personality, some of the qualities of the 7 will have emphasized the way in which he dealt with his fellow human beings in everyday life.

He was probably quite reserved toward others, and not interested in social and superficial relationships.

Interpersonal relationships were only important to him when they took place on the deeper level. In his youth, he may have been overly sensitive or shy. Although he was certainly kind and sensitive toward others, he was reserved in his private life, particularly during the years of youth. His basic nature was open to his surrounding world, and he was interested in how and why things are as they are.

The Horoscope of Mikao Usui

After I had enthusiastically read Dr. Usui's numerological analysis, the thought occurred to me to ask our friend Ginny Bydder, a Reiki teacher from New Zealand, to cast us a horoscope for Dr. Usui. I am not a great fan of horoscopes that place too much emphasis on the future and the past, mainly telling us when we marry, become rich or poor, die, or take a long journey. For me, the future is relatively uninteresting and the past is over. The only thing that we really have available to us is this moment. And astrology can be a wonderful aid to us in grasping this momentary reality of ours.

With its help, we can often very clearly illuminate abilities, talents, and behavior patterns, thereby making life easier for the respective individual or his loved ones.

The person of Mikao Usui is still a great mystery for many of us, and I would like to attempt bringing him closer to all of us with the help of the following horoscope. Unfortunately, since we still know little about his life, his personality, and his character, and the people he was close to have long died, I hope that we can attain a bit more clarity in this manner.

I have somewhat shortened the horoscope and brought it into its current form.

Mikao Usui was a man driven by a strong desire: he wanted to help humanity. He had a clear vision of his aims in life and of the transformation that would take place in Japanese society in the future. He may have had influential friends in politics who could have helped him positively influence the society. He had many interests, particularly in the areas of philosophy, religion, and spiritual knowledge and growth. Both life in the public limelight and the discovery of new paths were important to him. He was an unbelievably motivated, warmhearted man who knew how to fascinate the people around him with his humor, his wisdom, and his charisma. He was very interested in travel and foreign cultures. He enjoyed making decisions, was a diligent worker, and had an overall enormous strength of character.

Communicating with other people was one of his specialties. It was easy for him to find a common denominator with others—even if this concerned a larger group of people. He didn't like to work alone.

He was sincere and had a sunny character. In addition, he was a reliable friend and a warm and hearty advisor. It was important to him to belong to a group, as well as having the feeling of being loved and accepted.

The relationship to his family may have suffered discord at times.

His rational mind was sharp and critical. He tended to plan everything down to the smallest detail and examine all the possible aspects of a matter. In addition, he was a charismatic speaker. Superficial conversation did not interest him.

It was a pleasure for him to live and experience his own creativity.

Loyalty and trust were a necessity for him. He had a strong sense of justice.

His basic nature was critical, without being negative, and he had a special talent for sparking enthusiasm in others. He basically didn't find taking risks to be unpleasant. He had a strong urge for freedom and didn't let anyone constrain him.

He possibly had a conflict within himself between freedom and expansion, but once this was mastered he lived a healthy mixture of enthusiasm and structure. He also had the tendency to spend all his energies and reach for the spiritual stars. It's possible that he considered himself intellectually inadequate in comparison to others.

Personally, it was very important for him to express himself, find enjoyment in life, and fan the flames of joy and happiness within his own heart.

He had the ability of seeing, understanding, and sharing with his fellow human beings the connection between mental and physical health!

The Traditional Reiki Degrees

The traditional Japanese Reiki system is divided into several degrees.

The Sixth Degree, called Shoden, is the lowest (our First Degree).

In turn, it is divided into Loku-To (6th Degree), Go-To (5th Degree), Yon-To (4th Degree), and San-To (3rd Degree).

In order to learn these degrees, a person must meet up to four times a month with his teacher until the teacher is in agreement that this individual could move on to the next degree.

During these meetings, the person repeats the five Reiki principles and recites and sing Japanese waka poems. He listens to a lecture by the teacher, does a breathing exercise called Joshin Kokyuho, practices a method called Rei Ji, and receives an energy transmission called Rei Ju.

The next higher degree is called Okuden and is divided into two parts: Okuden-Zenki (first half) and Okuden-Koko (last half).

The symbols were taught in the first section. In the second part, distance healing and mental healing was learned. In addition, the methods that Dr. Usui talked about in the section in this book on "Questions and Answers" were taught.

The following degree is called Shinpiden and is only passed on to a very few chosen students by the Reiki teacher.

Once the student has been initiated into Shinpiden, he can receive the permission to professionally treat others.

Only someone who had completed the Shinpiden can become an assistant to the teacher. This position is called Shinan-Kaku. The word Shinan-Kaku means something like "teacher's assistant."

When the teacher considers it appropriate, he gives his student permission to hold his own meetings and have students of his own.

This position is called Shihan. The word Shihan means teacher. However, this term includes a feeling of authority, a role-model function, moral strength, and wisdom.

Authentic or Not Authentic

There is an old controversial issue in the Reiki community: the question about the "original" Reiki. What actually are the original methods, what has been changed for which reasons, and what has possibly improved since the time of Dr. Usui's death? Before I dedicate myself to this topic, I would like to once and for all clear away all the misunderstandings about the actual course of events after Dr. Usui's death:

As we know, Dr. Usui was the head of the Usui Reiki Gakkai (the Reiki organization that he had created himself). After his death, the chairmanship went to one of his closest friends, his colleague Mr. Ushida, who also wrote the inscription for Usui's memorial stone at the Saihoji Cemetery in Tokyo. Mr. Ushida was therefore Usui's successor. After Ushida's resignation, the next in the series of successors was Mr. Taketomi, who was followed by Mr. Watanabe, Mr. Wanami retired from her post in the beginning of 1998. The current president of the Usui Reiki Ryoho Gakkai is Mr. Kondoand Ms. Koyama, a charismatic lady in her nineties.

In Japan, there never has been a title like "Grand Master" or "Bearer of the Line."

However, Mr. Chujiro Hayashi, who was trained by Dr. Usui and, as an esteemed student, had the permission to have Reiki students of his own and train them, but was never appointed to be a successor to Usui. He was just one of many students who enjoyed this privilege.

In Japanese Reiki circles, very few people ever heard of Ms. Takata.

It's true that Mr. Hayashi operated a dojo (practice hall, school) in Shinano-Cho (Cho means town, Shi means large city) with ten beds available. According to reports by people at that time, these beds were always occupied. This statement apparently refers to the "Reiki clinic" that Mr. Hayashi was said to have run. But this is probably an imprecise translation of the Japanese word byoin, which is often falsely translated as clinic. Even a tiny doctor's practice is called by this word in Japanese.

When it is said in the West that there were many Reiki clinics in Japan during Usui's time, this probably refers to smaller establishments. We haven't been able to find one single hospital or one single larger clinic that has ever worked with Reiki. But I am certain that this fact will change in the next century.

At this point, I would like to quite emphatically say that I have nothing against Mr. Hayashi, Ms. Takata, and all those who came after them. I don't even know them! I am solely interested in the truth, as pleasant or unpleasant as it may be. I am convinced that Dr. Usui and his legitimate successors deserve the truth.

Many of us, including myself, probably have the tendency of just hearing what we want to hear and are capable of understanding. The work with Reiki power has naturally continued to develop and experience certain changes.

It's certain that every Reiki teacher instructs in his own way and changes the system so that it fits in with his personal approach and harmonizes with his personal understanding of it.

In both Reiki lines, but more in the Western system than the Japanese, there have been some enormous changes made. Many important aspects of Reiki work have been removed from the traditional system by either C. Hayashi or H. Takata. I don't know which of them made these changes, but they have also added many good things!

Now I would like to go into more detail about the social/ cultural and linguistic reasons for the differences in the Western and Eastern Reiki systems. Many of us find the Japanese to be mysterious, friendly but reserved, always smiling but still never cheerful. We almost always see them in groups, and it's difficult to make personal contact.

After years of experience in my language school, I have come to the conclusion that the East and the West differ fundamentally in their ways of thinking and feeling. For example, the Japanese mainly use their intuitive right brain hemisphere. In my opinion, the reason for this lies in the thousand-year evolution of the Japanese language, among other things. The Japanese characters, called kanji, are not sounds like the letters of our alphabet, but pictures. The kanji for mountain or river are wonderful examples of this.

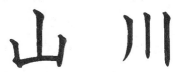

Kanji „Yama" (mountain) and „Kawa" (river)

This means the Japanese think in an abstract manner, in images from the days of childhood. Logic is not a topic of interest in Japan, and after almost seven years in Japan I only know two Japanese who (can) think logically and linearly. This isn't meant to be a valuation: the Japanese simply think in a different manner that is in no way worse than or inferior to our own. Intuitive thinking is a wonderful ability, and the world would be richer if Westerners would also master this art.

To spread the Japanese Reiki system, which is organized in a very intuitive manner, in a Western nation, it had to be divided into logical steps. The Reiki energy naturally didn't suffer as a result of this and whether the one system or the other is used doesn't matter at all.

In Western Reiki, the initiation rituals have been established in a very systematic manner. In the traditional Japanese Reiki, the teacher was permitted a great deal more freedom in following his inspiration. But it also wasn't simple to become a Reiki teacher, and only certain spiritually developed students were selected for this purpose. We could certainly argue about whether it's better to only train spiritually developed students to become Reiki teachers—but who wants to decide this point? In my career as a Reiki teacher, I have already experienced some surprises in both directions in this regard. Some of the students I had felt to be mature and integrated let the fact of being a Reiki teacher go to their heads; other students, who I considered to be sleepy and confused at the time, now often give me reason to thank them for their wise advice!

I think a detailed and time-tested initiation ritual is absolutely necessary in the West, where the Reiki Teacher Degree is freely available to anyone with the necessary small change. An initiation doesn't take place on its own through a book or video. A catalyzer, a teacher in this case, must always assist here.

On the other hand, the spiritual initiations of the enlightened are a completely different story that cannot be applied to Reiki initiations: spiritual masters like Jesus, Buddha, or Osho initiate thousands of people without knowing them individually, looking at them, or touching them, let alone speaking with them. To do this, the master no longer even has to be in his material body. But we don't want to become megalomanic: let's leave this up to the enlightened!

Twelve hand positions, which didn't exist in the Japanese system, have also been added to the system in the West. In the Japanese system, there are naturally also certain guidelines, but the hands are more or less given a freer rein in finding the places of the body that need to have energy directed to them. As we have personally seen in the texts with the questions and answers by Dr. Usui, the afflicted parts of the body can also be stroked, looked at, and breathed on in order to set the body's healing powers in motion.

I personally find the hand positions to be very helpful for beginners in particular since they direct energy to the entire body and at the same time connect both the patient and the treatment-giver to the Earth. Intuition is certainly an important tool, but it isn't all that harmless since the boundaries between intuition and illusion are quite hazy.

It may also be that Mr. Hayashi or Ms. Takata simply didn't understand the significance of some things or that the traditional methods couldn't be made compatible with the Christian slant that people wanted to give Reiki in the USA (and perhaps had to give it so that it would survive in a Christian society). We can imagine the situation shortly before and during the Second World War. It would have been absolutely impossible to propagate a Buddhist-oriented Japanese system of healing in America without getting into a tremendous amount of trouble as a result. Westerners would probably never have heard of Reiki had it been taught in its original state in Hawaii. I therefore thank H. Takata from my heart for opening the door to Reiki for us. However, in present times it's no longer necessary to depict Reiki as Christian. I have nothing against Christianity, but Dr. Usui was not a Christian.

The Japanese Reiki methods should now be taught and learned once again. It would be a pity to let them gather dust in the closet of secrecy.

Western Reiki students have been told that all the Reiki practitioners in Japan died during the Second World War. Of course, this is an absurd fairytale. The fact is that the Usui Reiki Gakkai had to frequently move during the war.

Since many of its members came from the ranks of the Imperial Marines, they had to be careful during the war to not be viewed and persecuted as part of the peace movement. For a while, the headquarters of the Usui Reiki Gakkai was in Togo Jinja, a Shinto shrine in Harajuku, Tokyo.

In Tokyo alone, there are at least four different "traditional" Reiki currents. The main line is still headed by Mr. Kondo. In the meantime, I have personally become acquainted with five different Japanese Reiki currents, which are spread throughout the entire country. Each of them has their own flavor and their own individuality. (In Japan, the Reiki that has been and is still practiced by Buddhist monks works with breathing and meditation exercises. Another source combines Reiki and macrobiotics. A third source combines Reiki and Shintoism, and so on and so forth.)

As far as I know, none of the traditional Japanese Reiki schools accept foreigners or Japanese who live in foreign countries into their circles. The headquarters under Ms. Koyama's direction was not interested in an exchange with non-Japanese. I can't blame them for this attitude after all the bad experiences that they have had with foreigners. Whether or not the winds will chang under the leadership of Mr. Kondo in this respect remains to be seen.

There are now thousands of Reiki teachers in Japan who teach the Western Reiki system. Since Chetna and I were the first to begin teaching all the Reiki degrees in Japan, many of them have either become acquainted with us or one of our students. Oddly enough, something that is imported back to Japan is often better received than something that has its origin in Japan and never left the country. The situation has been similar with macrobiotics.

The Western Reiki that is taught in Japan has with time absorbed many aspects of the New Age from its teachers and is therefore very similar to the Reiki known in the West. After they learned from us, some of the Japanese Reiki teachers learned from other teachers and connected several systems. Others mix Western and Japanese systems.

Reiki adapts to the abilities and interests of those who practice it. Why shouldn't it?

For me, in Reiki everything revolves around one axis, the axis of energy. And this energy is the same everywhere, no matter from what country, from which direction or philosophy it comes. Reiki energy is and remains Reiki energy without any attributes and without limitations. This certainly is a reason to celebrate!

Chapter 3

THE MENTAL BODY

SHARING

I have never understood why some Reiki teachers want to keep their knowledge to themselves. The same attitude has been found in the major religions of the world for thousands of years. In India, for example, the Brahmans kept their knowledge secret from the common people so that they could maintain their position as mediators between God and the rank and file. They even went so far as to develop a scholarly language, Sanskrit, for the most significant teachings, which was permitted to be learned by only one specific caste and not by women at all! In response to this, Gautama Buddha began teaching in Pali, a language of the common people. We can belatedly express our warmest thanks for this!

Knowledge that isn't shared with others stops being knowledge. The word needs someone to hear it in order to become a word. There are naturally things that should not be told to everyone, but this applies not only to Reiki! In my opinion, all the things that are currently being publicized on the Internet and in books about Reiki today go much too far. Although I don't consider it immoral to publish initiation rites and symbols, I do think it is pointless and senseless. This does not help anyone, even if it satisfies some people's curiosity.

Yet, when it comes to information that's important and interesting for all of us, I have a completely different opinion: The more we know about Dr. Usui and his methods of healing, as well as the healing methods that have been created during the course of time by other Reiki teachers, the more effectively we can all use Reiki. Reiki isn't dead matter and therefore constantly continues to develop with the help of thousands of Reiki teachers and students. Honoring the original Reiki methods is good and wonderful, but this does not mean that nothing new should be added to them.

A few days ago, I had a three-hour conversation on this topic with the well-known American Reiki teacher and author William Rand in the Shinkansen express train from Tokyo to Kyoto. He emphasized how important it is for a Reiki teacher to tell his students when teaching a method what he has added to it so that the basic teaching, as he learned it from his teacher, does not become diluted. This is why many Reiki teachers not only instruct Reiki One, Two, and Three (or Four), but also give advanced training courses that often consist of their own additions. This applies to my wife and me as well.

As I see it, it is important for each of us involved in Reiki to begin listening to our own inner voice and experiment with Reiki. Where would we be today if humanity had never continued to develop?

FEAR

Whenever I have an important decision to make or a strong desire besieges my consciousness, I ask myself what my motive might be. Using the distance-healing symbol of the Second Reiki Degree, I connect with my heart chakra, send the mental-healing symbol, and seal it with the power symbol. I breathe into the spiritual heart and ask about the reason for my wish. Absolute honesty with oneself is required at this point. If my motive should be fear, I don't follow the wish to its fulfillment. I thank my heart for the clarity attained and drop the wish. A neurotic wish analyzed in this way usually does not return. It simply dissolves.

Particularly when dealing with desires that are strongly charged emotionally, it may be better to ask your partner what he or she considers to be the motive. You can either do this in a conversation or by using another Reiki method: the partner sits on a chair and you stand behind him or her. Ground yourself with the power symbol or, if you have already learned Reiki Three, with the master symbol. Then draw the power symbol on the back of the partner's head with your finger. Let the energy flow and then draw the mental-healing symbol at the back of the partner's head at the point where the spinal column meets the back of the head. Once again, let the energy flow and seal it with the power symbol. Then step to the side of the partner, place one hand on his forehead and the other on the back of the head. Feel yourself to be like a hollow reed of bamboo, like a channel for the divine energy. Feel how white light streams through you from head to foot and let this light flow through your hands into the partner. Now ask your partner's higher consciousness what the reason is for the wish or the decision. Stay open for everything, whatever may happen now.

Thank your partner and give him a few minutes time to experience this beautiful state of mind before the two of you speak about your experience. It is possible that you—or even both of you—will have received suggestions from the higher consciousness, the inner wisdom that dwells within all of us. Now evaluate these together.

The way in which a therapist imparts insights to his client can immensely help or hinder the success of the therapy. If the therapist's words hit the client like a sledgehammer, the latter is certain to react defensively. The therapist then categorizes the client as resistant, and the client feels the therapist to be insensitive. The result is that both close off to the possibility of success.

I experience this sort of thing every day between parents and their children at our school. So it is important to be as sensitive as possible when you work with such subtle forms of therapy. Instead of "you are...," "it may be that..." or "could it be possible that..." are definitely more suitable.

Many of our desires are based in fear. For example, it is possible that someone wants to become rich because of an elementary fear of going hungry. Or that someone wants to remain poor because of a fear of change, fear of responsibility, or a fear of money! As you see, the reason for both of these cases can be the same. Decisions made on the basis of fear will never be freed from the energy of fear, and something affected by fear is and remains a poison for the soul.

What actually is fear? Fear is a mechanism of tension, the opposite of trust and openness, a sign that the ego does not want to let go of the self-created duality. With the help of the ego, we constantly mark the boundaries between ourselves and the surrounding world, insisting on our independence. I am this and that and can do this and that, and I do what I want to do. I, I, I! There is no room for mutuality, unity (in the sense of being one), and trust within this attitude.

The political and business worlds are much too willing to found their promises on a structure of fear because we all have such difficulty in liberating ourselves from our own fear. I personally am not the most courageous person in the world, but I believe that it is important to first become conscious of our own fears and face them head on. Once we look fear in the face, it will usually disappear on its own.

I remember an experience that I had a few years ago in India: Ever since my childhood, I have found snakes of any type to be unpleasant. One day, I filmed a performance by magicians on the street, as often can be seen in India. At the end of the show, one of the magicians finally coaxed his cobra out of its basket and asked me to come closer. He let his helper hold my video camera and wanted to place the snake around my neck. I felt a totally queasy feeling and wanted to avoid this experience, but the magician was not to be trifled with. He put the snake around my neck. After an initial restlessness, I began to relax and experience the beautiful creature in its peaceful nature. Even today, I can still laugh about the look on my face in the video. Not that I did not like snakes— I was simply afraid because I did not know what to think of them.

What we are unfamiliar with is what causes us to be afraid. And the unknown lurks in every moment. Who knows what may happen right now, tomorrow, or in ten years? Fear blocks and paralyzes us, makes our hearts bleed, and causes the intellect to become inflexible.

The power, greed for money, and lack of responsibility that has crept into Reiki—or the business with Reiki—during the course of the years are no different either. We cannot harmonize these problems when we hide from them and want to cut them to pieces because of our fear. The path of integration first goes through the peaceful confrontation within ourselves!

So let's think about what bothers us in relation to the way in which Reiki is passed on, how it is taught and sold. Then we will be on a constructive path.

In the final analysis, everything always boils down to working on ourselves. Teaching others is at best the second step.

POWER, MONEY, AND REIKI

Two things that become a lethal poison for the soul when they are mixed are certainly power and money. Knowing that in the West Reiki has not been spared of this poison makes my soul ache. In Japan, Reiki has nothing to do with money—it plays no role whatsoever. The dynamics of the morbid power struggle surrounding Dr. Usui's legacy, which we actually all share with each other no matter what corner of the world-wide Reiki family we are a part of, must first be understood so that we can drop it for once and for all.

This actually isn't a matter of who is fighting with or against whom—who the warriors are in this battle is completely insignificant. There's no point in portraying the people who try to possess Reiki for themselves as scapegoats and the cause of all evil. The desire to want to patent Reiki isn't a personal idea of an individual but a collective folly that has finally found an appropriate vehicle for its realization. If Ms. So-and-So had not done it, then someone else would certainly have come up with it.

An Indian saint by the name of Nisargadatta Maharaj once responded to the question of why he never spoke about the terrible circumstances of the Indian-Pakistani war: "Because you (the listeners) are both the murderers and the murdered." I often heard my master Osho say that only an enlightened person isn't a part of all the evil in the world because only an enlightened being is conscious of his/her actions.

Power mercilessly corrupts human beings. Once a person gets a taste of exercising power over others, he will have no other choice as long as his third chakra isn't completely balanced and centered. He will be carried away by the power as if it was a storm wave and lose himself within it, even if he rationalizes his actions time and again. I am certain that someone who has warmed up to the thought of monopolizing Reiki could find some good aspects to it. But this does not help the matter: Reiki, meaning life energy; is and remains as free as the wind, constantly accessible to us all, and someone who attempts to keep the life energy for himself is doomed to failure from the start.

Power in its primeval form is nothing other than energy, nothing other than strength. It always depends on how it is used. The same naturally applies to money as well. When both of these are only employed for the advantage of an individual or a small group, the result is always a catastrophe for the rest of humanity.

Money and power are interesting topics in relation to the spiritual world in particular. Many Reiki teachers bring little business and communications experience with them. They often exploit their power over their students in an unconscious way.

Of course, it always takes two players to play this game—the one who exercises the power and the other who gives up the power over himself to the other person. The victim and the aggressor form a symbiotic relationship. In almost every family, such role-playing takes place between the various family members. In my childhood, I was always the poor victim and my brother the evil aggressor—even if this was not the case and I had annoyed him!

Once more, consciousness is the key to happiness. At the moment that we become aware of our own power or that of the other person, the decision is obvious.

We all long for love and attention from other people. There are a great many different tricks for getting this attention. Being a powerful person is a path that appears to certainly lead us to our goal. Once we have a taste of what it is like to exercise power, it isn't easy to become a simple, apparently powerless person again. We should differentiate between power and strength here. It is possible to be a strong person without having to exercise power over others.

Especially in a spiritual realm like Reiki, exercising power is particularly harmful. I recommend every Reiki student to separate from a power-hungry Reiki teacher if the latter isn't willing to return to a loving state of light and unity. The spiritual ego is the most stubborn and unpleasant ego of all!

Power isn't something like our personal property. Instead, it is a collective feeling that has been given to all of us from the start. We begin to have a choice of whether or not we let this wave carry us away once we have become aware of it.

The collective unconscious sometimes guides entire cultures into the spiritual abyss. A situation that has repeatedly astonished me is the fact that often within a short span of time, several Hollywood films appear in the theaters with almost the same plot. For a time this may deal with intruders who threaten the "home sweet home" and the happy family, and then the topic becomes kidnapping, and so on and so forth.

What we call our own opinion, our own idea, our own goal, our own will is often just the collective unconscious that drives us in a certain direction. The path out of the darkness of the collective into the light of individuality is illuminated through spiritual awareness. This awareness does not just come to us through something like Reiki. Each of us must work on it for our entire lives. Through his initiation, a Reiki student or Reiki teacher receives a wonderful present from existence, but he must himself work on his own psychological maturation. There are certainly a great many misunderstandings related to this. A Reiki initiation does not make you holy or enlightened or better than other people. It simply opens a door.

Money is an inexhaustible topic. At the moment, I am sitting at an airport restaurant in Mumbai, India, drinking tea. In my wallet are 913 Indian rupees, 1500 Korean wong, 9000 Japanese yen, and 250 U.S. dollars, as well as a number of credit cards. The rupees will be enough for my dinner, the wong are for the subway from the airport in Seoul to the city, the yen will cover the distance I must travel in Japan, and the dollars are for a few presents to be purchased along the way. When I was a child, I loved playing Monopoly, and this is how my attitude toward money has remained. Its purpose is and remains something for us to play with. But there are a great many playing partners in this world who take it far too seriously.

An unbelievable amount of money is being earned everywhere with Reiki, resulting in a great deal of power. Many teachers who used to have very good earnings with Reiki must now share their earnings with countless other Reiki teachers. It is clear that this hurts. And I am in exactly the same situation! But because many of us are unwilling to deal with others in a civilized way, a conflict arises that unfortunately is carried out at the expense of the issue at hand, Reiki, in this case. A look at the advertisements in "New Age" magazines gives me a really strange feeling. Just a few days ago, I discovered someone in an Indian magazine who calls himself the "fourth Grand Master of Reiki." Because there are so many Reiki Masters, now we also need a Grand Master. Where should this all lead to?

I don't think that Reiki should be taught for free. Money is just a tool meant to more easily organize the exchange of things or services. The problem with money is of a psychological nature, and actually isn't related at all to money itself. Money is completely free of values. However, we associate it with certain feelings, ideas, and ideologies.

There are basically two separate camps: The one side considers money dirty and bad and believes that it will corrupt anyone who has it. It believes in love as its god and cannot bring love and money together. The other side chases after a steadily growing bank account throughout its lifetime and feels utter contempt toward the poor wretches on the other side. Love is only a means to an end here, to greater security. We know that many marriages break up because of money problems. Even in countless communes, whether spiritual or not, money leads to power struggles and other disagreements.

Ever since the days of childhood, we have all come into contact with our parents' money problems in one way or the other. Whether our family had too much or too little money at that time does not play the slightest role in this. The emotions attached to the money make it so difficult for us to deal with it.

I suggest that we give money back its original purpose as a tool and separate our feelings from it. This isn't to say that we should not be happy or annoyed about money. However, I do consider it helpful to become as clear as possible about our own motives for earning money and our own reactions in relation to money. Money is neither good nor evil.

As in all situations in life, it is important for each of us to find our own individual middle course. And this path of the middle demands absolute clarity. In order to help me achieve this clarity, Madhukar, a dear friend, gave me the following exercise some years ago: He asked me to write down everything in a notebook that came to my mind about money, both positive and negative. At our next meeting, he advised me to now record everything that I had ever heard my father, my mother, and other important people in my life say about money. It suddenly became clear to me that my thoughts about money were not based on my own experiences, my own opinion, my own fears but that all of this was simply the sum of my own conditioning. The whole house of cards collapsed as soon as light was shed on it. Within the few years that followed this experience, I found my own path in relation to money.

So what should a Reiki initiation or treatment cost? This question is very difficult to answer since it depends completely on the culture and the related social circumstances. It is extremely difficult to put a price tag on Reiki since we are completely different as individuals, as well as the situations we find ourselves in. One-hundred dollars may have exactly the same value for one person as one dollar does for another.

In our Western culture, we often don't sufficiently value something that has come to us with either no or little expenditure of energy. But the situation may be completely different in another culture. For example, I received a telephone call from New Zealand a few weeks ago from a Maori elder who has taught Reiki to her people for many years without charge. This immediately felt right to me. The motive is simply the most important thing.

I also know a wonderful healer in Austria who has people "pay" for his treatments with prayers. In Finland, the Finnish Reiki teacher Leila Anderssen recently told me, it is customary to "pay" the Reiki teacher part of the fee in social work instead of cash. So a Reiki student can give free Reiki treatments in a home for the aged or donate money to a relief organization. No limits are set on the imagination here.

What I understand to be much more important than money is that the student learns for himself, that the energetic relationship between the student and the teacher is balanced, and that both of them feel good about the agreed-upon exchange, whatever it may be.

REIKI SNARES

Time and again, I have seen how some Reiki teachers elevated the Reiki energy into a divinity and attempt to suddenly not let anymore "unspiritual" influences flow into their lives. Then they no longer drink tea or coffee, don't talk about the weather, only rely on their intuition, and have a "spiritual" explanation for every situation in life! Reiki is the only thing that exists, and the ground under their feet is suddenly gone.

For me, Reiki is a wonderful tool, but it is just one of the tools in my tool kit. In the final analysis, it always depends on the person using the tool and, above all, how the tool is used. If Reiki does not help bring more joy, more intensity, more harmony, more love, more wisdom, more openness, and more integrity into a person's life, perhaps it is the "wrong" tool or is being used "improperly." I don't mean this "wrong" in a technical way, but in a spiritual sense. If Reiki makes the Reiki channel arrogant and stubborn, then he is on the wrong track.

Since we often have a hard time evaluating ourselves, I suggest that you occasionally ask your partner or a good friend to give you a completely clear and honest "evaluation" about yourself: what you need to work on, what the other person sees as your problem area, where you stand in your own way, how you can further develop yourself, what positive changes have taken place, and if there is still a hitch somewhere. This topic brings to mind the eighth Waka poem by the Meiji Emperor. I was very impressed that an emperor could write a poem like this:

> *Being friends*
> *Being able to show*
> *Each other our errors*
> *Is the true shrine*
> *Of friendship*

At our house, the approach described above works wonderfully, and we both learn from each other every day as we gradually are able to free ourselves of our own arrogance, our narrow-mindedness, and all the other follies that we drag around with us.

If you don't know anyone in whom you can have this much trust, from the depths of my heart I hope that you soon meet someone with whom you can grow. To prepare yourself for this, imagine as precisely as possible what kind of person you would like to meet, including what he or she should look like, which character traits he or she should have, and so forth. We've being making very successful use of this approach for years in our language school when we look for a new teacher.

With this method, you can open your mind in a certain direction and the hoped-for person can enter your life. You're worth it!

SUFFERING

We practically inherit the willingness to suffer in our Christian culture, and there's actually nothing wrong with suffering once in a while. Suffering can intensify our empathy and sympathy for other people and their problems. But it is neither pleasant nor useful as a basic policy. Many of us have the opinion that we must suffer if we want to be alive, but I don't think that suffering is necessary for a happy life.

There is actually no such thing as suffering. When Gautama Buddha said that all life is suffering, he meant that being in an unconscious state is the same as suffering. Suffering is always our own evaluation of an unpleasant state. The fragrance of a rose, for example, can cause an asthmatic to suffer while the rose fragrance is a source of joy and inspiration for others.

We have a blind Reiki student, an impressive man who works as a masseur and acupuncturist. The last time I saw him a few weeks ago, I noticed that one of his fingernails was attacked by a fungus. It became quite clear to me that it does not matter to him at all since he cannot see it! I am not trying to say that we should not look at things, but that we give them the reality of their attributes of "good" or "bad," which actually don't exist.

Some of us feel more comfortable with suffering than with being happy. For about twenty years now, I have been professionally involved with many people and have noticed that there are individuals whose path in life constantly runs in and out of psychological and emotional suffering.

My situation is exactly the other way around. Since childhood, it has always been relatively easy to influence me with beauty and cheerfulness. An attractive woman, a pretty hand, a beautiful tree, a nice smile, and a happy song can easily cast a spell on me. Because I identify so much with happiness and beauty, or, let's say, with the idea of beauty, I place value upon how I act or how someone else acts, how he or she looks, and then easily get lost in immaterial things. Chetna is wonderfully amused time and again when I let myself get taken in by a smile.

So neither the one extreme nor the other is good when it isn't united with its opposite. We should therefore learn to accept life in its totality and live its counterpoles. A harmonious mixture of tears and laughter belongs to a fulfilled, intensive life. My master Osho once said to a Western student of his who had come to him because she was totally distraught about something that had happened: "Mukta, you cannot have the mountain peaks without the valleys."

EXPRESSING FEELINGS

I often heard my master Osho say that feelings must be brought to light in order for their purpose to become clear to us. The purpose of so-called negative feelings should be brought to light so that they can heal and the so-called positive feelings so that their light can spread even further.

Expressing our feelings is a balancing act at the start. Like tightrope-walkers on the circus rope, one tiny wrong movement to the left, right, upward, or downward is identical with falling into the depths. It isn't easy to share our feelings with someone close to us without pouring them over him and burying him beneath them.

The only way to learn how to gracefully express our own feelings is to practice doing so. Because it is often more difficult to express our feelings to people close to us, it is best to start with ourselves. Simply go for a walk or sit down alone in a quiet place and tell yourself how you feel about yourself. Then tell yourself how you feel about a person close to you without passing any kind of judgment on your feelings. There actually isn't any difference between the so-called "good" and "bad" feelings. The person who feels them is always the same!

When you have done this a few times, choose someone in whom you have total trust. Ask her or him to simply listen to you and then unconditionally pour out your heart. In a relationship, it often isn't easy to be honest because we say that we don't want to hurt the other person. I think this is true only to a limited extent. The rest of the truth is that we are afraid the other person would no longer love us if we express our feelings in their entirety. I recommend that you enter into a pact with your partner that allows both parties to be unconditionally open and honest. The reason why my wife and I are so close is probably because we don't have any kind of intimate secrets from each other.

In our language school, I have repeatedly noticed that it is often easier to express our feelings in a foreign language because we don't identify with it as closely. Perhaps this is why speaking a second language in the family makes our partnership even more harmonious!

But the simplest way is certainly just plain openness. By constantly being honest, we disassociate increasingly from our feelings. At the beginning, we may possibly swing from one extreme into the other like a pendulum and somewhat exaggerate the expression of emotions. It will become increasingly easy to share the "negative" feelings with time. After a while, it then becomes possible to speak about our feelings as if they were someone else's feelings.

THE INNER CHILD

Seen in the light, I think that it is an illusion to believe that the entire human being becomes an adult. Although we all get older, our body constantly grows and changes, but certain aspects of our psyche remain that of a small child. Modern psychotherapy and hypnotherapy speaks here of the so-called inner child. Osho often said that most people just become older instead of growing up.

I personally have precise memories of my childhood and the way in which my consciousness perceived its environment and itself. I basically have not changed! Even the childlike character traits have remained, although they have changed somewhat during the course of the years. Instead of Lego, soccer, Monopoly, and go-carts, my childlike interest is now attracted by CDs, computers, earning money, and cars.

In psychotherapy groups, we have often discovered in recent years that adults immediately begin to play like little children when given the opportunity. Our state of adulthood normally does not permit us to play without reservations, although we very much long to do so.

For me, the Reiki path includes the integration of all aspects of the character and personality. This also applies to the integration of the inner child. In order to connect with this portion of our self, I suggest that we make use of the magical Second Reiki Degree:

By using the distance-healing symbol, establish a connection with your inner child. Use the mental-healing symbol in order to heal this childhood situation and seal it all with the power symbol.

In case you have a hard time sensing the child within you, take a childhood photo as an aid and try to identify as intensely as possible with this picture. Try to remember the clothes you wore in the picture. Feel how your skin feels, how it smells, and how the colors affect you. The more you let your senses serve you, the better. Now try to remember your surroundings. Were you alone, together with friends, or with your family? Were you at home, at the playground, or on vacation with your parents? How did you feel on this day?

Now try to remember the feeling of your self, how you experienced yourself. Do you feel weak, strong, sad, healthy, cheerful, or perhaps even afraid? Perhaps you also just feel your energy.

Working through undigested childhood memories can bring quite a few things to light. Until I learned Reiki Two, I hardly had any memories of my early childhood. Just like the cork suddenly flies off a bottle of champagne, my conscious mind was suddenly swamped by a flood of memories.

It appears that time, and our past along with it, is suspended when it comes to our character. We are a conglomerate, the sum of our experiences from earliest childhood to the present day. All of our experiences, even if they lie in the past, are still present at this moment and influence our decisions. This means that in a mysterious way we live our entire lives during every moment. I am a child on the one level, a teenager on another level, and then an adult—and this all happens at the same time!

The reason why we want to drive the inner child out of our conscious mind is that a child is basically open and vulnerable. Every child probably wishes to finally become an adult so that it no longer is hit, punished, and humiliated. Once grown up, we discover with astonishment that the feelings beating within the child's heart can still be found within the adult's heart. They are probably even stronger than they were during childhood. Only one possibility of rescuing ourselves from feeling then remains: we suppress our feelings as much as possible. Yet, no problems have ever been solved by repressing them.

I will deal with the expression of feelings in greater detail in the next chapter.

Chapter 4

BEING FREE

CONDITIONING

The term conditioning implies that humans or animals are so imprinted through certain repetitive behavior structures in relation to specific processes that, even in their young years, they no longer have the freedom to determine their reactions to certain impulses. Conditioning takes place not only on an individual level, but also on the collective basis. It constantly hits us from all sides: from our society with all its rules and morals, from our native language with all of its subtleties, from our personal family situation, and naturally from the climate and geological zone in which we live.

One example of collective German conditioning would be, for example, that Germans always think they know everything better than anyone else!

Collective Japanese conditioning causes the Japanese person to smile and nod when someone asks if he understood something, even if he did not!

Another example of German linguistic conditioning is that every noun is given a gender, making it either masculine, feminine, or neutral. This means that speakers of German can never look at things without having reservations...

One example of Japanese linguistic conditions would be, for example, that the Japanese often avoid using personal pronouns when speaking about themselves or their group. This gives them and their friends the feeling of solidarity and unity.

I am not interested in using this to generalize the behavioral patterns of different cultures, but there are simply certain patterns that apply to almost every one of us, even if we find this to be unpleasant. The ego naturally does not want to hear about something like this since it will feel insulted in its honor as an independent being with its own freedom to act and its own free will. Unfortunately, we are not free.

The Armenian mystic George I. Gurdjieff spoke about humans as "food for the moon." I think he wanted to use this image to explain that the belief in a human being's personal will is an illusion. A student of Gurdjieff's, the well-known mathematician P. D. Ouspensky, explained the concept of conditioning with a clear analogy. In his book The Fourth Way, he spoke of humanity as if it were a group of people who find themselves in prison (conditioning, unconsciousness). In order to escape from this prison, they need help from the outside—help from someone who knows the prison well and is familiar with the possible paths of flight. Alone, without a spiritual master (meaning someone who had previously also been unconscious himself but is now liberated from the prison) or a group of seekers, he says, a flight from the unconscious is virtually completely impossible. This is primarily the case because we are not even aware that we are in prison, and cannot be aware of it.

The nature of conditioning is like a continuously repeating tape, constantly playing in our unconscious mind without our knowledge. According to its definition, something unconscious—meaning a process that takes place in the mind without our knowledge and our control—is invisible for us. So we need someone else to hold up the mirror so that we can see our own conditioning. We could now argue that no one could know us better than we ourselves, but the nature of conditioning means that we cannot see it on our own.

For me personally, it is an immense help to live with my wife, who comes from another cultural group. Time and again, we point out the rigid mechanics of our way of thinking to each other and therefore have the opportunity of growing beyond our limitations. At the beginning of our relationship, we naturally also had terrible misunderstandings because each of us did not understand the other person's conditioning, let alone really comprehend it. But when there is an understanding of another culture, the exchange between people of various countries and cultures can be even more intensive.

This means that it is easier for someone from England to see the conditioning of a German, and my individual conditioning is more apparent to my wife or another person who is close to me than to myself. The result of this is that we easily feel attacked when someone reminds us of our lack of freedom. But this does not help at all. The path to freedom does not always lead through a rose garden, and pain is a good teacher!

The first time when someone points out our painful lack of freedom to us, we must have enormous trust in him since we are not capable of seeing our automatic reactions. For me, this trusted person was my master, Osho, and I am eternally thankful to him for making me aware of my unconscious state at that time.

Conditioning could be called the programming of our brain. Our brain is the computer and our way of thinking, with the limitations mentioned above, is the software. In order to achieve more freedom of action beyond this obstacle, the programming must only be seen with clear eyes. Seeing something with clear eyes means not assessing it, not judging it, but simply seeing it as it is. By seeing clearly, the identification is broken and the conditioning loses its power, the power of unconsciousness.

Once we are able to see like this, the possibilities that can be chosen reveal themselves. We must no longer show a specific reaction and can decide whether we want to become annoyed, sad, or nervous—or not. This state of not having to react brings us into the present, beyond the future and the past, into a meditative state.

THE POWER OF THOUGHTS

We all have heard Berthold Brecht's remark that "thoughts are free." If we want to consider this remark in its entire significance, we must first take a look at what thoughts actually are. What we call our self, our personality, is actually nothing more than a chaotic conglomerate of individual thoughts. So this means that a thought represents only a fraction of our personality. Interestingly enough, our self therefore consists of a vast quantity of disconnected thoughts, which are all born of the past. This present moment, the only moment in which we actually are alive and can experience, does not include the past and the future.

There are two types of thoughts. The first type goes on its own dream journeys without any activity on our part and without our control, taking us along whether we want to go or not. The second type is conscious thought. Both types of thoughts cannot be censored, stopped, or changed by others. Thoughts are things in a form that isn't yet solid and crystallized. It isn't hard for us to move things from one place to another, and this fact does not cause us any difficulties. But the same also applies to thoughts. They have no boundaries set for them and they move completely unhindered through time and space without resistance. This fact brings certain implications with it.

The first implication is: be careful about what you think. A thought that constantly repeats itself in our heads, lurks around, takes on its own life in time, and a continually repeating vibration in the more subtle worlds lets it take on a physical form of its own. This is the reason that so-called "positive thinking," auto-suggestion and hypnosis, when used often enough, produce good results. But we must therefore be very careful about what we put into our subconscious mind. It is a torment to work with a computer that has been poorly or improperly programmed.

We should be particularly cautious with thoughts that affect others. If we think badly about someone else, these fine vibrations reach this person and have a negative influence on him. In most cases, this occurs in an unconscious way on our part, but this does not mean that the negative thoughts will diminish in their effects. The more sensitive an individual becomes to the energy of the whole, the more he will also feel the negative aspects.

I've heard time and again that it isn't possible to send negative energy with Reiki. I would like to agree with this in principle, but someone who consciously attempts to influence others in a negative way will also abuse Reiki for this purpose. There isn't anything in the world that is just "good," because good and bad are attributes that we human being give to things.

The more clear, and therefore stronger, the developing person becomes, the more dangerous he will basically be. He can harm himself and others. It is important for him to learn to control his thoughts and, above all, never lose respect and compassion toward all living beings.

Using an example from everyday life, I would like to explain in more detail how we unconsciously send bad energy to others: Imagine that you're sitting in a car and a pedestrian crosses a red light in front of you. If you are relaxed and in a good mood, you simply take your foot off the gas and that takes care of the matter. If you are nervous or in a bad mood, you become annoyed and maybe swear to yourself. If the pedestrian presses a button at the signal and forces you to stop as a result, you will also be angry at him. However, the energy of your aggravation does not just stay with you in the car, but also influences the pedestrian as much as it does you. This occurred to me for the first time as I crossed at the signal in a meditative state a few months ago and suddenly soaked up the annoyance of a driver. This experience has made me a more peaceful driver!

We naturally just cannot drive negative thoughts out of our heads, and I also don't want to suggest here that they should be suppressed. Paying attention to them is important: once we become aware of the negativity, we have the choice of letting them go.

Negative thoughts radiate a strong power of attraction for us, which is why there are many exercises for training the power of thoughts in a positive way in Tibetan Buddhism. One exercise from The Tibetan Book of Life and Death by Sogyal Rinpoche is described on page 99 in the chapter "My Reiki Path."

It has been said that the positive thoughts of an enlightened soul can help the recipient on his spiritual journey. This is why the blessing of a master in any form is considered so important everywhere in the world, whether it is given to a human being, an animal, nature, or even a machine.

Exactly the same thing happens with Reiki. By means of the Reiki symbols, the energy is concentrated on a specific point, whether this is a person or thing, and radiated there. So when we want to transfer healing or blessing to another person, it is important to formulate our thoughts as precisely as possible so that the desired effect can occur.

One of our friends, for example, uses the Reiki symbol with unbelievable success in her vegetable garden. With the distance-healing symbol, she sends energy and specific instructions to all the plants in her garden and harvests three times as many vegetables as her neighbors.

The radiating or sending of energy and thoughts also functions without Reiki symbols. So it isn't necessary to wait for the Second Reiki Degree in order to "send" energy or your blessing. I am familiar with a Reiki current in Japan that does not use the symbols even for distance Reiki healing.

If you can perfectly focus your mind, then they are probably superfluous. However, the symbols are wonderful tools for us beginners: who among us would try pressing a nail into the wall with his hand when he has a hammer at his disposal?

In keeping with our experiences, practice also makes perfect here. The more we use the Reiki symbols and focus our thoughts, the greater will be the success that occurs as a result.

SPIRITUAL AWARENESS

In this chapter I would like to describe how we can learn to observe the inner dialog that stops us from living in the present. This observation is meditation. We don't need psychotherapy or any other technique in order to change ourselves, to grow, and to develop. All of these therapy methods work with the psyche, which naturally is imperfect and can be improved. Consciousness is perfect as it is and needs neither growth nor change. In the words of J. Krishnamurti, "the observer is the observed." If this is so, then we have actually already reached the end of our journey.

Spiritual awareness isn't like an ability with which we are born, but the ability to learn this is something we all bring into the world with us. However, most of us don't look in this direction. Spiritual awareness must be trained like a muscle, and this training is harder than any kind of physical training will ever be.

We can try testing the status of our watchfulness with a short exercise:

Sit down in front of a clock and look at the second hand with as much concentration as possible. You will see that you probably become immersed in your own thoughts within a few moments and completely forget the second hand.

Indian philosophy claims that if we would just spend 48 minutes in a state without any thoughts, we would become enlightened. This sounds inconceivably simple, but after the above exercise you will see how difficult it is to not be carried away by your thoughts for even one minute.

Thinking in itself isn't the problem. Without the ability to think, life would be a torment and today we would still be sitting like the apes in the jungle. Some of us may argue that it perhaps would be better that way. There certainly would be less mischief taking place on the global level if this was true. But let's return to the concept of thought: The problem of mental activity isn't thinking itself but the compulsion to think that does not give us a moment's rest. What we normally call thinking is actually nothing of the sort. We jump from one thought to the next like apes in the jungle and completely lose ourselves in what happens around us. We therefore constantly sacrifice the present for a dream world that we have built for ourselves. While we eat, we mentally go shopping, and when we go shopping, we are already eating in our thoughts! It is a crazy world, and I am certain that a Martian would consider us to be totally off our rocker with our incessant compulsion to think. Pure or clear thinking is something completely different, so I will not go into it at this point.

I would just like to talk about the spaces between the individual thoughts here. Let's first look at the nature of the mind and the thoughts. Since we can observe our thoughts, we can say that the mind and the thoughts are two different things. My meditation teacher Osho explained the nature of the mind with the following analogy: the mind sees the thoughts like someone looking at a film in the movie theater. The film (the thoughts) is projected onto the screen (true existence) by the projector (the mind) and interpreted to be the truth. So what normally happens in our thought processes is that we identify with our thoughts, understand the film to be true life, and forget true existence, at least for a while. This is also exactly what happens at the cinema, and a good film is one that spellbinds the viewers and takes them away from reality.

We identify with a dream figure projected onto the screen and travel through a series of different emotional states. We become afraid when the hero is attacked in the darkness by an evil person with a knife, and we sincerely amuse ourselves when something funny happens, and, in another situation, our heart becomes heavy with sadness.

Somewhere in his writings, Tolstoy told of how his mother was so deeply moved by the plot of a play at the theater while the coachman who had brought her there froze to death in front of the theater. This is precisely how we act with our own life! Through our daydreams, we are put into a trance-like state in which we feel good, bad, or normal.

So how can we free ourselves from the non-stop current of the inner dialog?

I have personally tried out some possibilities:

Reiki
During self-treatment or the treatment of another person, you can use Reiki to direct energy to yourself and thereby put yourself into a state of intensified awareness. With each hand position, you not only let the energy flow, but also the awareness. It is helpful to breathe into each of the twelve hand positions or the seven chakra positions while you give the treatment. The breath is the bridge to consciousness. It is often helpful to adapt your breathing rhythm to that of the recipient.

Mantras and prayers
With mantras and prayers, the mind is focused on a specific thought, and it isn't permitted to go off on its usual dream journey. As a result, a pleasant calm is created on the one hand; yet, on the other hand, the mind is also put into a tensed state through this manipulation, and I don't find tension to be natural.

Lao Tzu, the original father of Taoism, advises us to be like water and go with the flow of life. There are naturally many paths that lead to more quality in life and awareness. Mantras should only be used under the direction of a competent teacher since, in working with subtle vibrations, they are capable of creating powerful changes. Prayers are safe, but I am not all that familiar with them.

Awareness exercises
When I first was at Osho's ashram in the Indian city of Poona about 19 years ago, we did a wonderful exercise during a psychotherapy group. With a partner, we went into the overcrowd-

ed streets of the city, a chaos of trucks, cars, motorcycles, rickshaws, bicycles, people, cows, water buffalo, goats, an occasional elephant, and dogs, all of which intertwined with each other in a completely unregulated way like fireworks, maneuvering with a sometimes tremendous tempo through the burning heat. While we walked through this confusion, we were to alternate with each other in repeating a certain pattern of meaningless words such as "ungolo mongolo, ungolo mongolo." The partner was to respond to this with "ungolo mongolo, ungolo mongolo." The magic formula was then repeated three, four, or five times and responded to by the partner. Even after just a few minutes of this exercise, I noticed that no other thoughts could gain a foothold in my brain, and my body maneuvered through the masses practically on its own, swiftly, and without ever running into anything. The exercise also brought with it an intensified level of consciousness, limited to that period of time. But who can just be occupied with "ungolo mongolo" all day long?

The Armenian mystic G. I. Gurdjieff gave the name of "self-remembrance"—being reminded of yourself—to what I call spiritual awareness. In order to help his students understand how to remember themselves, he asked them, for example, to always remember themselves whenever they passed through a door.

I sometimes write myself little notes that I attach to strategically important places such as the refrigerator door or the dashboard of my car. When I still smoked, I used to put notes with suggestions like "I am in the here and now" or simply "I am" into my box of cigarettes. You can tailor this type of exercise to yourself. However, the problem with this exercise is that it loses its benefits with time. As soon as the mind has adjusted to it, it no longer brings the desired result. More consciousness always leads to results. The more aware we become, it is only logical that unconsciousness will decrease. Unconscious actions like the excessive consumption of alcohol, cigarettes, and other substances will increasingly fade into the background. It is no longer necessary to want to forget the present with the help of a bottle of wine if we want to try to live every moment consciously. (However, I don't consider the consumption of alcohol, cigarettes, coffee, and the like to be immoral.)

Hypnosis and auto-suggestion

These two methods can become excellent tools on our path, but they require a relatively intensive amount of effort. Auto-suggestion must be constantly repeated so that it functions, and a trained therapist is required for hypnosis if you are not well-versed in self-hypnosis.

Be extremely careful when putting suggestions into your subconscious mind. Once the worm is in the apple, it isn't all that easy to remove it again!

Meditation

In my opinion, meditation is by far the best method. During meditation, we learn to observe the inner dialog without manipulating it in any way. We don't try to chase off the thoughts but look at them like a film within us.

There are many different types of meditation, suitable for the various types of people. In many of these, the key to awareness lies in the breathing. Observe your breathing and you will automatically be looking at your thoughts, emotions, and physical sensations.

For meditations like Vipassana or Zazen, it is certainly helpful at the start to retreat to a quiet place. However, meditating for half-an-hour or even an hour daily is just one drop on the hot stone of everyday life.

The great thing about a breathing meditation similar to the Vipassana is that we can become immersed in it during practically any kind of activity and only during activity. This is an old Hindu meditation, a sutra that can be found in a wonderful book by Paul Reps.* It is said to have been given by the Indian god Shiva to his beloved Parvati. Unfortunately, a detailed explanation of this meditation can only be found in Osho's book Vigyan Bhairav Tantra, which is currently out of print. I think this is one of the best books available on meditation.

The sutra says:

"When involved in worldly activity, keep attentive between two breaths, and so practicing, in a few days be born anew".

---

*Paul Reps, Zen Flesh Zen Bones, Charles E. Tuttle Company, ISBN 0-8048-0644-6

With the help of this meditation, you can experience everyday life with all its activities in a deep state of awareness, no matter whether you go for a walk, read a book, or watch television. In my opinion, the most important thing about any type of meditation exercise is that it helps center the person who meditates. Our consciousness is normally not concentrated. Only in the moment in which we concentrate it on a certain point can we constructively use it for our growth.

The more intensively we become involved with meditation, the more we separate ourselves from identifying with the inner dialog. The result of this is that we become less dependent upon our thoughts and feelings, moods, and physical well-being or lack thereof. This in turn results in an attitude of trust in the present, a feeling of the appropriateness of everything that happens or does not happen.

This does not mean to say that we should stop following our impulses and no longer open the umbrella in the rain. To the contrary, we learn to act more effectively because the mind is clear and the thoughts can act in an independent manner.

In a world like ours in which hardly anyone can afford to spend a lifetime with meditation in a cave, this type of "meditation in the market place" is the loveliest present you can give yourself.

TRANSIENCE

All things are transient in our earthly existence. Health and illness, happiness and sadness, poverty and wealth are opposites that complement each other. One cannot exist without the other.

The only thing that we can be absolutely sure of on earth is death. All living beings must at one time or another die, must shed their mortal bodies, their memories, abilities, thoughts, feelings, knowledge, leaving their earthly achievements behind them and dissolve in eternity.

The Japanese Zen master Kozan Ichikyo wrote the following poem in the year 1360 before he laid down his calligraphy brush and left the world while sitting upright:

With empty hands I came into this world
Barefoot I leave it
My coming and my going
Two simple events
Interwoven with each other

We not only come into this world and leave this world alone, we also cannot take anything along with us into the other world—in case there is one. If there is no permanence, it is also nonsense to tie our boat to our possessions and dreams. Consequently, it is also senseless to cling to certain philosophies, thoughts, feelings, and values, which we take along to the grave when all is said and done. But instead of taking them to the grave with us, it is possible to already learn to let go of them during our lifetime. I think that this is a task in life!

This moment is the only moment that we truly have available to us. Tomorrow exists only in our fantasy, and yesterday is also just a thought, a memory that cannot be relived. We are totally free and unattached at this moment. At their core, our life philosophy and our ideologies are insubstantial soap bubbles, a toy for human beings.

This may sound somewhat fatalistic, but it isn't meant to be at all. Absolute freedom brings absolute responsibility with it. Not only are we responsible for our actions, but also for our thoughts and feelings. Every stone thrown into the sea of collective being forms a little wave that sets itself forth through the entire universe.

Part of our responsibility as a human being is taking care of both our planet and our earthly body. Many mystics have said that only on the Earth is it possible to become enlightened in a human body. We all too easily forget the importance of our earthly body and treat it without respect. It is written in the Bible that God created human beings in His own image. We should try to see ourselves in this way from today on: we are the manifestation of the divine here on the Earth. And this divinity is the only thing that survives life and death in the light of eternity.

Chapter 5

EXPERIENCING

EXPERIMENTS WITH REIKI

People often ask me whether they are permitted to do this and that with Reiki. Each time I am astonished that there are Reiki teachers who downright prohibit their students to experiment with Reiki. The only thing that I find ethically indefensible is sending Reiki to someone who has not asked for it. In my eyes, this borders on manipulation, although the other person isn't harmed by it. However, we should not injure another human being's freedom. Several years before I got involved in Reiki, I had an unpleasant experience when someone sent me Reiki energy without my knowledge and consent. I had felt manipulated and "not myself". A few years later, I found out what had happened ...

The only exception I make in this respect is when I see an ambulance going to the scene of an accident or to a hospital. With the help of the distance-healing symbol, the mental-healing symbol, and finally the power symbol, I send energy to the situation, praying that enough energy for the healing or whatever is necessary may be provided by existence. Even in this situation, I don't send Reiki to the injured person directly.

Each of us goes our own way. Just like no two snowflakes are the same, we are all different from each other in a wondrous manner. What is good and advisable for one person can be uninteresting and even harmful for the other. I therefore advise all of you to experiment with Reiki and find out for yourself how Reiki can help you advance in your own life. There is nothing that we cannot do and are not permitted to do when we ask our hearts to be our advisor. No teacher can teach this to a student because you are the only one who ultimately knows what is good for you.

Not only for personal reasons, but for the sake of the Reiki power, I consider it important to do experiments. Life constantly moves forward. If Reiki does not continue to develop with us, it will soon land in the storeroom as a rusty tool. If Dr. Usui had not experimented, there would not be any Reiki at all today! I know many people who practice Reiki and never really use their abilities because they are afraid of doing something wrong. What a waste of time and energy that is!

In order to get the stone rolling, ask your subconscious mind to tell you the ways and techniques for using Reiki, that you had not been aware of up to now. It is certainly possible that even with Reiki a personal aversion or incompatibility can come to light. For example, it may be that a certain symbol does not harmonize with a specific part of the body or organ. If at some point you don't feel well during or after one of your experiments, you can break off the contact with the symbols by intensely rubbing your hands together or washing your hands and arms up to the elbows with cold water. If this still does not do it, then gargle with cold water, take a shower, and, while under the shower, repeat a short prayer, a mantra, or an affirmation related to well-being, or simply sing a song. Taking a walk is also a good technique for some of us to separate from something unpleasant and bring the energy back to the essential.

REIKI AND OTHER LIVING BEINGS

Reiki energy isn't just reserved for human beings. It surrounds and flows through human beings, animals, trees, stones, the oceans, and the air. The human being also isn't the only living being that seeks and needs healing in our unhealthy world. As we have read in the chapter on "Questions and Answers," Dr. Usui said animals also have the ability to heal. This become clear to me intuitively about four years ago. I initiated Tao, our black-and-white cat, into Reiki at that time. I felt like a blasphemous fool, but Tao liked the initiation. If I happen to have a stomachache once in a while, I ask her to stretch out on my belly. This is how our entire expanded family gives each other treatments.

Since her initiation, she has been exemplary as a healthy cat and has never fought with the other cats in the neighborhood since then, even though she spends her days outside in good weather. There also were not any battles when we moved two years ago and she had to establish a new territory. We arrogant human beings certainly could learn some things in this respect. Yet, despite all this, Tao has not turned into a vegetarian: some birds and mice still fall victim to our Reiki cat.

Is it immoral, desecrating, or blasphemous to initiate an animal? I don't believe so, as long as you feel yourself to be a Reiki channel and not the "Creator." In the words of my friend and Reiki teacher Ginny Bydder, the student isn't initiated by the Reiki teacher, but through him. So the Reiki energy isn't given to us by another person, but already belongs to every living being from birth on.

I have already heard of many cats who settle in the lap of the recipient during an initiation or other energy work, even if they usually were not all that interested in cuddling. Why should it be kept from them?

Nature with all its living beings should be seen as a whole, and I consider it a great foolishness of humans to place themselves above all the other living beings. I feel that the most delicate plant and the tiniest ant is just as worthy of respect as the biggest elephant and the holiest person! This isn't a philosophy but a feeling that has grown within me during the course of the years. I am certainly not a saint in God's eyes: as a child I enjoyed torturing and killing birds, fish, insects, and other animals. I liked to fish, and killing and removing the insides of the catch did not bother me at all. Today I feel badly if I even drive by a butcher shop in my car!

The key experience that let me become a vegetarian happened in 1977 in Ireland. I was hitchhiking through the country with a few friends, and we lived in a tent on a farm for a week or two there. The farmer had loaned me his shotgun, and I went off to hunt rabbits. When I finally saw a rabbit sitting in the sun, I aimed the gun, suppressed the humane feeling that flickered within me for a moment, and—boom—a piece of dead meat was laying in front of me.

Even weeks after that, I was plagued by the picture of the pink rabbit ears that had shone so wonderfully in the sun until I had sent them to kingdom come together with their owner. I felt miserable and inhumane in the truest sense of the word.

My cruelty had so filled me with consternation that on the very day I was initiated into Reiki Two, I connected myself with this situation and in tears, apologized to the Creation for my atrocity.

Until I met the Reiki teacher Christel Seligmann in January of 1998 in Germany, the topic of Reiki initiations for animals was still unpleasant for me and I was reluctant to speak about it in public. I found out that she had written an entire book about her experiences with Reiki and animals and became enthused about it. I can warmly recommend it in particular for veterinarians and those of us who live out in the country or have pets.

TIME TO EXPERIENCE

Reiki has recently been offered everywhere as a quick course. I call this the "just-add-water" method, which is meant to create a wonderful Reiki menu within the shortest amount of time.

I can very well understand that we are all in a hurry and always want to have everything as quickly as possible, but I believe that it is better to take as much time as possible in approaching the various Reiki degrees. This amount of time is different for each individual. I don't want to make any rules about it since there are enough of them already!

I have heard that no more than two days should pass between the initiations of the First Degree since the energy would otherwise go up in smoke. In the old days, people met once a month for six months here in Japan in order to learn the First Degree. We teach it either on one or two days, which can also be a week apart.

There are various ways of teaching the Second Degree. Some teachers initiate once during the Second Degree, and others do it three times. The three initiations can either be divided over three weeks, which gives the student much more time to experience the Reiki power and to experience the individual symbols or, if only one initiation is done, just teach the students one symbol a week.

Our friend Shizuko Akimoto, a wonderful healer to whom we must give thanks for much of the news about Reiki that I have publicized, recently told my wife on the telephone that each of the Reiki degrees has a specific value. If Reiki One and Two are taught too quickly after each other, the value of the First Degree isn't properly grasped and this means casting pearls before the swine. But I don't believe that anything can be done wrong or destroyed with rapid Reiki training.

It may also be necessary to teach someone the entire Reiki system or a large part of it within a short amount of time, particularly when this person is seriously ill. For example, I personally received my first Reiki initiation in a single week and then bombarded my teacher on the telephone with questions for months afterward. In the meantime, I have learned various systems.

Reiki itself, meaning the energy, cannot be taught. It reveals itself completely on its own if we are attentive. And this attention is what the teacher promotes in the student.

ENERGY

It would be a joke to want to say something about energy itself and explain it to someone who does not feel it. It simply must be experienced. Some people would say that they are not sensitive enough to feel energy, but this certainly isn't entirely true. Each of us feels the energy that surrounds us in our own individual way. Some of us feel energy, while others see or hear energy.

I often think about the way in which energy reveals itself, changes, and how it moves. In physics, it is said that energy is never lost and can never be lost, even if it changes its form. Water either becomes steam or ice when it is drastically heated or frozen. Cooled-off love may turn into hate or apathy.

We normally feel better in the presence of an energetic, positive person than in the presence of someone who is hanging in the ropes without any energy. We often feel drained, in a bad mood, and empty after being with such people.

Every feeling, every emotional state bears a certain energy within itself, and we "feel" this energy. When we go home and notice when we come in that our partner isn't feeling well today, we feel this person's energy. If we feel ill at ease time and again in a certain café, then it is probably the energy of the place that puts us off. The more sensitive we are in terms of energy, the more careful we will be in selecting the places where we go. Growth isn't always just a piece of cake: we not only gain new friends and insights but also lose old friends and habits.

There is an enormous difference between the dynamics of energy and the dynamics of a savings account. (Here I am not talking about money as energy but about the dynamics of hoarding.) In the savings account, the more we leave the money alone, the more quickly it multiplies. However, energy only multiplies when we use it, share it with others, and let it move freely. Stagnated energy is similar to an empty savings account and brings its owner even more out of balance. As a result, it is important that energy is kept in motion, whether this concerns a business transaction or your own body.

The Reiki power within us can be of service in both instances. When we treat ourselves or other people, the energy is set into motion on all levels and the recipient's energy household comes back into its natural state of equilibrium.

Learning to sense energy in our own way is certainly helpful, as long as we don't forget that even the energy flowing through us and around us is just a phenomenon. I have noticed that the energy flow within, as well as in the outside world, is given much too much attention in New Age circles.

It is always important to see who feels the energy—who is it that feels the current of energy, observes it, enjoys it, or is swept away by it? Who has the experiences? The Indian saint Ramana Maharashi (1879—1950) recommended that his students constantly ask themselves "who am I?" as a form of meditation. Who is it that hears, sees, feels, tastes, smells, speaks, is healthy or sick, is born and dies? Only when we focus our attention in this direction will Reiki work become work on ourselves. Only then it will become a spiritual path.

GROUNDING

When you are dealing with any type of energy work, it is absolutely necessary to be solidly rooted with the Earth. And Reiki is certainly no exception here. In general terms, men are in greater danger than women: they more easily get lost in their own thoughts and inspirations, thereby confusing reality and imagination with each other. Because of their natural mother instinct, women are already more closely connected with the Earth. It is no wonder that we speak of Mother Earth. Just being together and living with a female partner often helps a man become more grounded.

The simplest way to ground yourself is perhaps physical work, whereby it does not really matter what you do. Whether you clean the house, paint it, do the gardening or carpentry work, work brings the consciousness that has moved into the more subtle channels through energy work back into the body and therefore to the Earth. If we would not need our bodies for grounding, nature would not have outfitted us with them on our path!

The crucial point regarding work is to experience every movement, every motion, as consciously as possible, to experience every stroke of the paintbrush as intensively as possible. Sports like bike-riding, swimming, or jogging that get the heart going and make us sweat are extremely helpful. You should naturally talk to your doctor about them beforehand in case your health isn't the best.

For men who live alone and men who are predisposed toward drifting off into the clouds, I would recommend doing certain grounding exercises on a daily basis if they cannot or don't want to engage in any physical work. Finding your equilibrium between heaven and Earth is a wonderful task.

Grounding with Reiki

Sit down on a chair with your feet parallel to each other or stand in a relaxed way on the ground. If possible, do this outside under the open sky. Now place both hands on your hara (energy point three fingers below your navel) and leave them there for at least ten minutes while you let your breath move deeply in and out from your belly. Feel yourself connected with your inner center and feel the energy from the Earth rise up within you until it reaches your hara.

Grounding can be done in an even more effective way with the power symbol. Draw the power symbol in any way that you wish and then send it first into both of your foot chakras, then to the hara, and finally into both hand chakras. If you want to ground another person, touch the parts of the body mentioned above and let the power symbol flow with the desire for grounding. For most of us, this grounding usually feels like the creation of a magnetic field, a tingling, or a pleasant sense of becoming heavier.

Connecting yourself with the Earth

You can connect yourself with the Earth in a wonderful way by laying completely stretched out on your back, either on your bed or the floor, and imagine that a type of root leads down deep into the Earth from your hara. Feel the strength and the nourishing energy from the inside of the Earth rising up into you.

Or feel yourself to be like a tree and imagine how the Earth protects and nourishes you with its forces.

Trees

Trees are concentrated, grounded energies that easily transfer themselves to us. This is why many of us like to sit under trees in the yard and let ourselves be charged with their energies, usually unconsciously.

"Sitting under a tree" also appears to be related to meditation. Not only my master Osho and Gautama Buddha, but also many other saints experienced enlightenment under a tree.

We can benefit from the help of the trees by either sitting in their shade, leaning on their trunk, or even embracing them. The first time you embrace a tree from the bottom of your heart may be a comical adventure, but you will stop feeling totally crazy after a few more times. I personally use my breath in order to intensify the absorption of the tree's energy. If you sit under a tree or embrace it, imagine that you draw in its energy into yourself with every breath. Then thank the tree for its generosity.

Autogenic training

An effective method of grounding, which I already described in greater detail in my book, The Reiki Fire , is the autogenic training developed by the Berlin neurologist Professor Dr. J. H. Schultz. There are a many good books available on this topic in the bookshops and a rich offering of courses.

Personally, I would always prefer to learn from an individual instead of a book.

FEELING GOOD

We all want to feel good, and an enormous amount of money is spent in this world in the hunt for well-being. A bigger car, a new apartment, a new dress, and a new partner—all of our wishes ultimately strive to let us enjoy our lives and ourselves. Something that is outside of us, which can be found in the world, naturally cannot bring us eternal happiness. Happiness can neither be found on the outside, nor is the happiness experienced there permanently. Life is a constant process of change, like the play of the tides or the succession of spring, summer, fall, and winter.

Even the Reiki power isn't an exception here. Although Reiki flows through us, as well as through everything else in the world, it isn't a magic pill that we just have to swallow to reach seventh heaven. A Reiki initiation is certain not to bring permanent bliss with it, and this isn't even the issue at hand. Earthly life consists of light and darkness, and the point is to learn to enjoy both of them as intensively as possible. If we would always feel well, we would probably die of boredom or ask the Creation for a serving of suffering!

It isn't my intention to say that we should stop longing for well-being since this is the most natural thing in the world. A Reiki session is so particularly pleasant for us because it brings us into an extremely agreeable state of consciousness. Many types of massage, yoga, and qigong, as well as listening to music, going for a walk, and having sex bring us into a state similar to that of a Reiki session. Through the monotony of the motions, the lightness of the music, or perhaps the pleasant warmth of the hands and the touching of the body, so-called endogenes (natural opiates) are formed within our body that put us into a blissful, trance-like mood. This mood naturally cannot be maintained throughout the entire day, since we otherwise would not get anything else done on the one hand and our power of sensation would ultimately be subdued on the other hand. Just imagine having to listen to a piece of music that you very much love throughout the entire day: after a few hours, you would probably either be ready to destroy the CD player or you would have completely suppressed the music out of your consciousness and practically no longer hear it.

So we should first learn to feel our body with complete intensity, in whatever state it may be. Simply close your eyes and feel how your hands rest on your knees and the warmth from the hands is drawn into the legs. Feel your back on the backrest of the chair, your feet on the floor, your breath as it moves in and out of you. At the same time, try to be totally free of judgment. Simply experience your body as it feels at this moment and try not to change your feeling. If a part of your body is tense, simply feel the tension. If you have pain, feel the pain without judging it. If a part of the body feels sore, then simply feel the soreness.

When you have practiced this for a while, try to deal with your thoughts and feelings in exactly the same manner. Experience them without wanting to change them and you will see that all at once you have suddenly become more independent.

You are neither your body nor your thoughts nor your feelings. You are the light of eternity, the breath of the universe. You are the Reiki power!

Chapter 6

BODY AND SOUL

BEING HEALTHY AND BEING SICK

It is neither good nor bad to be healthy or sick. The (conscious) being that experiences health or illness is always the same. It never changes, even if it takes on one form or the other for a time.

Most of us naturally find the first state to be more pleasant than the second. But a so-called illness also has some positive aspects to it. In this way, the body announces to us that we have neglected to take proper care of it or that it needs rest in order to balance itself again. I don't know if there are actually always psychological reasons when a person becomes seriously ill. In New Age circles it is commonly thought that every health disorder has a certain emotional, mental, or psychological basis. I consider this theory to be only partly true and I would like to look at it from a different point of view. This attitude is probably more the rational mind of human beings believing that it will lose its predominance over people's inner life and now must simply find an explanation. When this has been found, the entire matter is stuffed into a cubbyhole of the memory, and we can heave a sigh of relief. Ah—once again, a puzzle has been solved, a secret aired!

But not everything can be explained in a logical way: try explaining a rose to a Martian! This simply cannot be done without experiencing it through sight, touch, and smell. I therefore personally tend to see the human being with all his weaknesses and strengths, as well as the universe that surrounds him, as a unity.

An interesting book on this topic is The Holographic Universe: "The World in a New Dimension" by Michael Talbot (Harper Perennial Library, ISBN 0060922583). In this book, Talbot gives an example cited by the American physicist David Bohm in his book Causality and Chance in Modern Physics.

Bohm says that even in science the causality for a certain effect is explained in a very biased way. He gives the following example: Can we say that the American president Lincoln was killed solely by the bullet of his murderer? Certainly not! There is an entire list of reasons to be given, beginning with the human being's physical ability of holding a weapon, to the invention of the weapon, up to the development in which the murderer learned to hate Abraham Lincoln, and so on and so forth.

The body, the environment in which it lives, the time, the family, social, and economic circumstances, the genotype, the season—in brief, everything plays a role in the physical, emotional, and psychological state of every human being. No healing can take place when the human being is divided into certain parts. Healing is always a process of becoming whole.

To claim that a person has an earache because he does not want to hear something is probably quite inappropriate. There are things that each of us don't want to hear! And this also functions without an earache.

I think it's simply outrageous to tell someone who is dying of cancer that he or she caused the cancer even if there might be a bit of truth to the idea. If you have ever experienced what it means to hold a friend dying of cancer in your arms during the last hours, you will certainly agree with me here. As if the disease itself isn't hard enough to cope with. Things look different if the sick person understands the misterious interrelations that may have created a favorable breeding ground for a disease to florish in.

I certainly would not make children who are born with AIDS or other still terminal diseases responsible for them.

Not only normal earthly mortals get sick and die of completely common diseases: Gautama Buddha died of food poisoning, Ramana Maharshi and Ramakrishna Parmhansa of cancer. My master Osho had asthma and diabetes, J. Krishnamurti was plagued by terrible headaches throughout his life, G. I. Gurdjieff and Meher Baba has serious traffic accidents.

Western and Eastern philosophies say that enlightened beings become sick because they take on the suffering of humankind. In my experience, everyone carries his or her own cross. The Indian mystic Meher Baba said somewhere that not diseases cause a person to die, but death! This sounds unbelievably banal, and I still remember precisely the situation as I read this: I had to laugh terribly hard, and only after a few days did I become aware of the depth of this statement.

My feeling is that illness and health are simply conditions that alternate with each other at certain intervals of time, often without any reasons that we can understand rationally or from an enormous variety of reasons. We are healthy for a time, then we become ill, and then we recuperate again. During the course of the millennia, we have learned to classify certain physical states as "good" or "bad." And here, in my opinion, lies the problem. Health and illness are value-free in their nature; like the two sides of a coin. Yet, we always search for the reasons for just one side of the coin, the illness. When we are healthy, we don't bother to ask why this is so: it simply is. So we should first learn to accept both sides as they are. This does not mean simply accepting your illness, going into a dark chamber, and wasting away. It means quite the opposite. Once the moral identification with the badness of the disease is broken, we are truly capable of doing something for our health. And when the body has actually reached the end of its journey, then it is possible to let go of it with gratitude.

It isn't my intention to claim that there are no physical, emotional, mental, or psychological reasons for specific illnesses. Sometimes these are so apparent that they cannot be denied. In exactly the same way, psychological disorders can also result from the physical level.

My theory is that body and soul cannot be divided. They are a unity, and an illness takes place on all levels at the same time. Since the subtle bodies are responsible for our thoughts, feelings, and energy supply and experience a constant exchange of energy and information with the material body through the chakras, meridians, and nadis, the interplay between the body, mind, and emotions is obvious.

This state of simultaneousness also applies to what we call time: feelings, thoughts, and the traumas that we encountered yesterday perhaps still gnaw within us today. Our memory not only takes place in our brain, but also in each individual cell of the body. These memories, particularly if they are of a traumatic nature, can remain awake in the cell memory for an entire lifetime. Cranio-sacral therapy, an apparently simple type of body work, is particularly well-suited for removing such trauma from the cells and bringing the cells back into a harmonious state.

It is said that there are so-called karmic diseases, diseases that only disappear when they have done their karmic duty. In this case, I think it would be better to completely set aside such theories as long as we don't understand their existential meaning. Most of us, myself included, don't have the competence for such an evaluation.

It is also possible that healing takes place through detours, the so-called healing crises. A healing crisis is a state in which a chronic disease is thrown into an acute state and can thereby worsen temporarily. The cause of a healing crisis is often the temporarily increased toxicity of the blood or of the lymph, which cannot be coped with by the excretory organs of the intestines, the liver, the lungs, the kidneys, and the skin pores.

There is no doubt that we can learn from our illnesses. I myself have been plagued since childhood by psoriasis, which has caused me to look at certain things with my inner eye. In times of stress, the condition wells up and shows me the necessity of relaxing. As a result, it has become increasingly clear to me how dependent I am on the opinion of others. When my skin has reddened, I feel slightly insecure, vulnerable, and afraid that other people may not like me because of it. During the course of the years, I have tried everything possible to get rid of this disease. My path has gone from orthodox medicine to hypnosis, psychotherapy, meditation, autogenic training, affirmations, faith healing, clairvoyance, homeopathy, Reiki, qigong, courses of treatment at spas, fasting treatments, up to self-treatment with urine, which brings very positive results.

However, a person must be quite desperate to start all of this!

In order to keep the body healthy, it is particularly important to pay attention to your nutrition. According to the nutritional researcher Dr. Bircher-Benner, "nutrition is not the highest thing in life, but it is the breeding ground upon which the highest can flourish or spoil."

The entire animal world is more intelligent in terms of nutrition than human beings. During the course of the millennia, we have lost the direct relationship to our body and no longer know what is good for us. It isn't possible to abuse our bodies for years without damaging them. The simplest way to find out what is good for you and what isn't is to be particularly attentive after you have eaten.

If you feel listless or nervous and want to go to sleep right away, then the food probably has not agreed with you. If you really want to know what benefits you, then write a journal for three months. In the finest detail, write down what you have had at each meal and how you felt afterward. Every morning, write down how you slept, how you feel, what your skin looks like, how your digestion is, and so forth. If you want to get more involved with this topic, I recommend the "Spiritual Nutrition and the Rainbow Diet" by Dr. Gabriel Cousens, M. D. (Cassandra Press, ISBN 069-1587520).

Seen in psychological terms, we very much identify with our body, so much that this is even shown clearly in our language. We say: "I am sick," not "my body is sick." Strangely enough, this identification with the body stops for most of us when it comes to maintaining its optimal health.

If you do become ill at some time, then treat your body in an especially loving way. It is easy to hate our own body if it does not function in the way we imagine it should. But only the opposite attitude is helpful and healing. When the body has been weakened, it needs even more attention than when it is healthy and strong. The part of the body that is sick needs loving energy. The mystic Rudolf Steiner said somewhere that we must love a disease if we want to heal it.

With the help of the Reiki symbols, it is possible for us to come even more deeply in contact with our body and mind.

In "From Medication to Meditation", (C. W. Damiel Company LTD, ISBN 0-85207-280-5) my master Osho speaks of how we can connect with our brain and ask it to give a specific message to the body. He says that it is important to not directly connect with the disease because then, I believe, it will even be intensified.

I suggest that you connect with the distant-healing symbol, repeat the symbol's mantra three times, and appeal to your brain. Then send the mental-healing symbol and seal it with the power symbol. Now ask your brain to tell the specific part of your body that the respective illness has fulfilled its purpose and can now fade away. Do this every day for one week. In the case of a chronic illness, do it for three months.

ACTIVATE THE HEALING POWER OF YOUR BODY

Disease isn't healed by a healer or a medicine that you take. With the help of the tools mentioned above, it is repaired by the body itself. Yet, the healing power of the body can be activated by many types of support.

The simplest and most important method is wanting to become truly healthy in the first place. This may sound crazy, but we are all attached in some way to our complaints and the opinions about them. If a person believes, for example, that the cancer tumor in his stomach is incurable, then he will certainly die of it. I have a few friends who have separated from so-called incurable diseases, but only because of their untiring zeal and discipline.

An important initial step is to intellectually and emotionally distance yourself from "your" illness—no longer called it your headache, your rheumatism, or your depression. Even just the act of separating from the identification alone will make life somewhat easier. The divine light that shines from within each of us is actually completely independent of disease, of good and evil. If we succeed in directing our attention from the disease to the divine, we will have come a giant step closer to being healthy. This type of spiritual self-assurance gives us a constant surge of energy, which we can then use to heal our bodies.

The "knowledge" that we have acquired starting in childhood often hinders us in the healing. It can actually be proved that much of what is offered to us as general knowledge is incorrect. An example of this is the opinion that we will catch a cold if we go outside with wet hair. The truth is that a cold is triggered by a virus, in a weak immune system but not from the combination of wet hair and going outside. If we become ill, we should definitely take a closer look at the opinions that we have about certain health disorders and disease in itself.

There are basically no limits set for us here on Earth. We always create them for ourselves. Fortunately, we have the possibility of dissolving these limitations time and again, no matter whether they are of a personal, social, cultural, religious, emotional, or intellectual nature. Hypnosis can provide a valuable service for us in this respect.

The first step to health and the activation of the body's own healing powers is always permitting your body to have enough rest, taking good care of it, and not waiting until you are over-exerted, drained, and ultimately become sick. This is a bit of advice I should pay more attention to myself! But as the saying so aptly states: Stupidity knows no limits! Unfortunately, we often only learn when we feel bad.

It is natural that the body changes with time and can no longer put up with as much as it did during the younger years. Eating habits also change. We require a clear attentiveness on our part to notice these fine changes and adapt to them.

The first time I had lunch with my wife in the ashram at Poona, the fork almost fell out of my hand when I saw what she had dished onto her plate, despite her slender figure: I had considered myself to be a glutton, but I had a child's portion on my plate in comparison to hers. She was thirty years old at the time, and within the next few years we suddenly both just ate half as much as before. Our metabolism had readjusted from 500 grams of pasta for lunch to 250 grams. Fortunately, we were aware of this change in our bodies and did not end up bursting at the seams as a result!

We should always observe our bodies with awareness and listen to its wishes and desires for change. The simplest method of listening to your body is to ask it before each meal what it wants to eat now. The trick to this method isn't to think about it, but simply pay attention to the first thing that comes to mind, even if this means a lot of work in preparation or going shopping for it.

But aging also has its advantages. The body and, above all, the mind, become increasingly sensitive and more receptive. In no case would I like to go back to "the good old days"!

Relaxation

If you want to or have to work a great deal because of external circumstances, it is important to take the highest quality breaks—to relax, meditate, go to the movies, or whatever else serves as relaxation for you. What is relaxing for one individual drives the next person crazy, which is why each of us has to find out for ourselves what works well. Fortunately, relaxation is an open book for someone who practices Reiki—if we can just remember how important relaxation is!

After relaxation, the next step is meditation as described in greater detail in the section on "Spiritual Awareness." Relaxation rests the body and the mind, but meditation relaxes both and the soul as well. And all good things come in threes!

Hypnosis

As high-quality tools, hypnosis and NLP (Neuro-Linguistic Programming) appear wherever spiritual growth, health, and harmony are involved. In my book, The Reiki Fire, I already described how we can create our own affirmations and learn the lower level of autogenic training. You can also use these techniques to strengthen the immune system and activate the body's own healing powers by either having yourself hypnotized by a qualified therapist or doing it yourself. When creating an affirmation, just be sure that it is always kept in a positive format, and that it makes you free. An affirmation or post-hypnotic suggestion that is limited in some way will only lead us into another, newly furnished dungeon.

Visualization

Since hypnosis either requires a therapist or at least a good bit of work on ourselves if we want to do it alone, I suggest that you start with simple visualization exercises. If you (like me) are not very visually oriented, this isn't as easy as it sounds. But it is fun to expand your own horizons.

Imagine down to the smallest detail how your immune system is bursting with strength and effectiveness, and the healing power of your body watches over your health like a good spirit. It does not matter how and what exactly you visualize as long as it provides you with light, strength, and self-confidence. If you have a Christian background, you can imagine a group of angels promoting your health. I personally envision an inexhaustible source of golden light that floods through me and enriches all the cells with powers of resistance. An army of miniature power symbols would certainly also be a great help for our visualized internal healing power.

Totally omit the concept of illness from the visualization. Illness is an emotionally-charged word and can have negative or intensifying effects on the health disorder.

Reiki

The inner energy circulation is intensified through the subtle energy channels as a result of the Reiki initiation. However, the ability to absorb energy from the cosmos is increased at the same time. So we can say that Reiki affects us from all sides, from within and without. In this way, it helps us once again achieve a harmonious, healthy equilibrium. The body becomes more resistant and has more of its own healing power available to it.

It has often been said that Reiki does not need to be practiced, that it is always there. It is naturally true on the one hand that the Reiki power is practically in our bones since birth. But, on the other hand, we and many other Reiki teachers have discovered that Reiki students often have more energy than Reiki teachers because they give themselves Reiki every day! So the flow of energy becomes stronger with practice since the Reiki channel is virtually "cleaned out" as a result of the frequency with which Reiki flows through it.

Body work

In addition to Reiki, there are also countless types of body work that activate the body's own healing power. Of the well-known methods, I personally prefer acupuncture, rebalancing, colorpuncture, and cranio-sacral therapy.

Chapter 7

MY PERSONAL EXPERIENCE

MY REIKI PATH

In the following chapter, you will find a report on my personal experiences with Reiki. Since my mind functions analytically, I have divided the experiences into seven parts. The number has no further specific meaning here.

Please don't expect that the same things will happen to you on your path as they did to me. It would be terrible if life would be so predictable. Although we are all made out of the same substance, of love, light, consciousness, or whatever you care to call it, our individual path is absolutely unique. In a mysterious and wonderful way, we are all different from each other and yet still the same. In the entire world, in the past and the future, there is no other person like you, with your wonderful body, with all your abilities, as well as your weaknesses. Let us celebrate this wonder of the human soul together!

Since Reiki is so interwoven with meditation and other growth processes in my life, it is difficult to decide whether certain experiences are based on my Reiki initiation. It is probably more accurate to say that they can be attributed to the entirety of my personal development.

After I had learned Reiki at the end of 1992 in Germany to promote my personal growth, I returned to Japan where I headed a language school, among other things, together with my wife Chetna.

Although I had a great deal of experience with meditation, psychotherapy, and body work, I knew little about energy work and healing. I had the opinion that energy work was reserved for a spiritual master who knows exactly to which physical and emotional states he wants to draw the students' attention, when he intervenes with healing, and where he lets life take its natural course. Today, I no longer see energy work in such a narrow way and simply consider it one of the greatest ways to share ourselves and the energy that flows through us with our fellow human beings.

Healing, I thought, is a gift given just to a chosen few healers. In a certain sense, this is still my opinion today, although every person is transformed into a "little healer" after the Reiki initiation. At that time, I considered myself to be insensitive in relation to energy and the subtle world, and I enjoyed making fun of those who worshipped crystals, channeled, and saw spirits. Seven of my twelve astrological signs are Earth signs: I love being rooted deep in the Earth with both feet, digging up the garden, and chopping wood. Yet, or particularly because of this, I decided to experiment a bit and enlighten my consciousness in this previously dark corner.

Chetna's background was completely different. After she, like me, had become a student of the Indian meditation master Osho, she learned many Eastern methods of healing in order to get rid of a hellish lumbago at the beginning of the Eighties. Among other things, she learned shiatsu, then a healing method from H. Noguchi, called Noguchi Seitai, and trained with the healer and qigong master Ishii, who was very well known in Japan at that time. Unfortunately, he died several years ago. Mr. Ishii initiated her into the art of healing and spurred her on to develop her own healing method because of her talent. She worked for years and refined this method, but did not teach it. At the end of 1997, she was finally ready and began to train her first students.

Chetna had often seen beings from other worlds, but oddly enough, these apparitions stopped the moment she met me! I have never been certain whether I should be happy or unhappy about that.

Shortly after my return to Japan, I initiated Chetna into Reiki in January of 1993. Although I actually had not planned to teach Reiki, after a few months we decided to offer all the Reiki degrees in Sapporo. We quickly discovered what is perhaps the greatest advantage of Reiki over other healing methods: the practitioner does not become dependent on the therapist, treats himself, and thereby gives himself the love and energy that ultimately heals him. In this way, an individual literally begins to take the responsibility for his own body and his own existence into his own hands.

94

We decided that we did not want to make our clients dependent on our healing powers and would prefer to teach Reiki. We naturally continue to give ourselves treatments, even up to this date. We encouraged our students to heal themselves. It is so easy to pass on the responsibility for your own body to a physician or therapist, even though it sometimes is necessary to do so. Always giving up the responsibility for one's own life has never helped anyone enjoy life. Our unhappiness always has its source within ourselves.

Since we were the first Reiki teachers of the Western line to permanently live and teach in Japan, we had to give some thought to how much money we wanted to accept for a Reiki initiation. We decided to pass on the entire knowledge to anyone who wanted it in order for Reiki to spread quickly in Japan and become accessible to as many people as possible in this way. The prices, particularly for the Teacher's Degree in the USA and partly in Europe as well, were so shamefully high in comparison to what was actually being offered. I don't mean to say that some courses of Reiki training are not worth their price, but many of them—including the cheap ones—unfortunately are not.

We thought about the matter for a few weeks and then decided, with an eye on the buying power of the yen, the average income in Japan, to offer Reiki One, Two, Three, and the Teacher's Degree for a total of 330,000 yen (about $2500). This not only included the Reiki initiations, but also our time, love, experience, attitude, and possible later consultations. We wanted to make Reiki affordable for everyone, but it also should not be too cheap. We wanted our students to honestly ask themselves whether they wanted to invest a larger sum of money, meaning a lot of energy, into their own growth. Once they made this decision, they would certainly treat themselves with Reiki and learn to value what they learned for the rest of their lives. Seen in this light, whatever you pay for a Reiki initiation is just a minor amount. When I consider how much money I have shelled out for cigarettes, beer, and wine...

These prices have remained the standard in Japan, although some of our students in Tokyo have lowered their prices in order to beat the "competition."

The first step

The first thing that I became aware of as a freshly initiated Reiki teacher was that the time difference between Germany and Japan was no problem for me. During the flight, I had treated myself with Reiki Two and Three. I arrived totally fresh in Japan.

This made me think that I would probably never become sick again, and then I promptly came down with a cold like I had never known before: for three entire months my body was virtually out of action! I believe that this cold represented a phase of deep cleansing and healing for the body and soul. Until then, I had mainly lived on the level of emotions and thoughts, and now I finally began to discover my body. I had used it like a lifeless machine, without loving it and respecting it, for thirty years. I took the body for granted and thought that it did not need to be taken care of lovingly.

However, the path to my body first led back to my youth. During this initial Reiki time, I worked by means of Reiki Two (distance-healing symbol, who/where/what, mental-healing symbol, power symbol, letting energy flow) on my childhood and spent countless nights on the sofa in the living room crying a storm tide of tears. Long-forgotten and even suppressed memories flooded back into my consciousness. I suddenly saw the battles with "friends" and "enemies" and all the mean things that I had done to other children and animals as closely and vividly as if it all were just yesterday. As the crowning event, I found myself confronted with a girlfriend's suicide, for which I had felt responsible to a certain degree. So I lay on the sofa at night and let all of this drift to the surface.

Healing and integration are impossible in the darkness of the subconscious mind. As in my case, memories spiced with emotions only apparently disappear, but they continue to silently and unnoticeably have an effect in the subconscious mind. Unfortunately, what we then call our own freedom of actions is then actually in truth just the undigested past that dictates our current ways of behaving.

The interesting thing is that at that time I never experienced myself to be suffering and never judged what I was going through as bad. It was clear to me that integration can only be achieved with empty hands, meaning without any still painful remnants of the past. In addition, the developing feeling of becoming whole brought an enormous strength and self-assurance with it.

With Reiki Two in turn, I apologized to those beings for my mistakes and stupid things I had done at their expense: by first drawing the distance-healing symbol, repeating the name of the person, the situation, and the time, asking forgiveness and sending the mental-healing symbol, and then finally closing the whole thing with the power symbol. I felt refreshed and like newborn. Some of the stones had fallen from my heart, the largest stone of which was that of the pent-up guilt feelings.

I certainly could have done some things in my life better, but now I also learned to finally accept myself as I am and my past as it was, without wanting to change anything about it. Wanting to change things often occurs from an egocentric dissatisfaction with the here and now, which actually has nothing wrong with it. The world is always in order in the here and now.

In April of 1993, we initiated the first group of four friends into the First Reiki Degree. Both of us were joyfully surprised by the energy set free during the initiations and in the course of the day. Although we had already treated each other with energy before our Reiki days, it appears that energy always flows so intensely between partners that it isn't possible to clearly define the boundaries between the two people and is hard to feel the energy of "the other." After the first initiation, the smiles never left our faces for the rest of the day.

We experienced our next surprise when we went to eat with our friends that evening. They all devoured their meal like a horde of hungry cannibals after a fast. But Chetna, who served us all the delicious meal, could hardly put a bite of it into her own mouth.

I immediately remembered the energy work that I had experienced between 1979 and 1981 in India. At that time, Osho gave energy transmissions every evening at his ashram in Poona, offering many of his students a taste of the divine. Afterward, a good meal and an Indian cigarette always brought me down to Earth.

Once people got a taste of the initiations, things suddenly moved virtually on their own. People hungry for Reiki, who had learned the first two degrees elsewhere, came from all parts of Japan to us in Sapporo. Up to that time, just Reiki One and Two had been offered by the other Reiki teachers.

We soon discovered that the so-called spiritual world was something different than the very holy idealism with which I had viewed it. Power and money appeared to be of more importance than love, light, peace, and bliss. I guess that happens even in the best of families.

One day, I noticed something strange: a wound that I got during the garden work just would not heal. Contrary to our habits, Chetna and I were nervous and imbalanced for two weeks. Our business had stopped growing: the telephone was deathly still and no one appeared to be interested in learning English or Reiki. Up to now, we had always had a lot of do and the sudden forced vacation made us worry.

When we took a closer look at our nervousness, we discovered that it did not even have anything to do with us. I immediately called my teacher in Germany and told him how we felt. Without giving it any further thought, he said that someone was manipulating us. The idea that someone wished us evil shocked me deeply. Up to this day in my life, I had always been convinced of the goodness in every human being. I believed that each person is basically good within his heart and that we all love each other in the depths of our souls. A new window opened for me, and when I think back to that time, I am happy that my horizon expanded, even if it hurt at first. It became increasingly clear to me that I was living in a romantic dream, miles removed from reality, that I had created for myself through the years and had learned to love. Reality was grinning at me with a frightening grimace.

My teacher was not at all astonished and told me that he and some of his other students had had similar experiences at the start. Dealing with this situation is part of the Reiki training, and we have to learn to cope with it. He promised that he would neutralize this outside energy and explained to me how I could protect myself in the future if I wanted to prevent such situations. Then he sent me energy on the telephone, and I immediately came to myself.

We both felt immensely relieved, light and full of joy. The moment I put down the telephone, our business rose from the dead. The same day, we received three new students for English classes and two people registered for Reiki. The wound an my finger healed the following night!

Since this experience, we protect ourselves from psychic attacks. I am familiar with several methods of protection. These include prayer, talismans, and Tibetan Buddhist techniques like the following from "The Tibetan Book of Living and Dying", by Sogyal Rinpoche (HarperSan Francisco, ISBN 0-06-250793-1):

Tonglen for Others
Imagine someone to whom you feel very close, particularly someone who is suffering and in pain. As you breathe in, imagine you take in all their suffering and pain with compassion, and as you breathe out, send your warmth, healing, love, joy, and happiness streaming out to them.

Now, just as in the practice of loving kindness, gradually widen the circle of your compassion to embrace first other people whom you also feel very close to, then those whom you feel indifferent about, then those you dislike or have difficulty with, then even those whom you feel are actively monstrous and cruel. Allow your compassion to become universal, and to fold in its embrace all sentient beings, all beings, in fact, without any exception: Sentient beings are as limitless as the whole of space: *May they each effortlessly realize the nature of their mind, And may every single being of all the six realms, who has each been in one life or another my father or mouth. Attain all together the ground of primordial perfection.*

There is also a wonderful Reiki method taught to me by my friend Walter Lübeck. Using the distance-healing symbol, connect yourself with your navel chakra and connect with your inner child. Ask your inner child to transform the negative energies that it receives into positive energy, send it the mental-healing symbol, and then close the whole process with the power symbol.

The second step
For about one year, we had been searching with little result for the origin of Reiki and researching Dr. Usui's tracks. Now we finally had success. Although we had found a direct relative of Dr. Usui's, the wife of his grandson, in 1993, she unfortunately had little to say about her husband's grandfather. It sounded

as if Dr. Usui had had a falling out with his family or at least one part of it.

One of our students who lived in Tokyo had found the grave of Dr. Usui at the Saihoji Temple on our behalf. A few days later, we heard from one of our students that a lady living in Tokyo had supposedly been practising Reiki since her youth. At that time, it was not clear to us that this was the rightful successor to Dr. Usui, Mrs. Koyama.

I had almost given up with further research and actually had come to doubt the historical figure of Mikao Usui. Had he actually existed or had he perhaps lived and worked under another name? The stories in the books and from Western Reiki teachers that were told about him were simply unbelievable, often even ludicrous for a person like me who thinks in a halfway straightforward manner. I also could not believe that in Japan, the country of Reiki's origins, there were no people who practiced Reiki.

I was practically thunderstruck for a while after hearing about Mrs. Koyama. Chetna spoke with her on the telephone and, for the first time in our career as Reiki teachers, we came to know the truth about Dr. Usui.

A whole new view of things opened up, but in order not to completely frighten us, life always provided just as many new revelations as we could digest at any moment.

Up to now, the importance of the word "Sensei" in Japan had not been clear to me. It means "teacher" and bears witness to the respect for someone who introduces others into his art. This may be cabinet-making, medicine, art—in short, any conceivable field. Chetna and I had always found it embarrassing to be addressed with this title, which is why we asked all of our students, even the youngest, to call us by our first names. It was apparent to us that this title creates a gap that is almost impossible to bridge between two or more people, which does not permit a heart-to-heart connection to arise. Seen in cultural terms, this Japanese word may have fulfilled its purpose in an authoritarian society, but we considered it to be outdated and out of place today.

In the so-called spiritual world, the "Sensei" title appeared to be even more desirable. During our first Reiki year, many people came to us who were mainly interested in the title, the power, and the income that would result from it—but not in their own development.

The Reiki Master title was, although now affordable for everyone, seen as a spiritual achievement and some of the newly baked Reiki teachers floated a few kilometres above the rest of us mortals with their halo in seventh heaven. We often wanted to give up Reiki once and for all because of this and turn our backs to the New Age world.

Although the business world is partly based on greed for money, power, and the inexhaustible drive for one's own advantage, at least the lines are clearly drawn. People basically follow the rules and many business people help each other in a very human way instead of fighting each other like the Reiki teachers do.

The culmination of this chapter and the process of learning about the human psyche surprised me in the spring of 1994 as several new Reiki students brought a letter to us in Sapporo written by one of our former students in Tokyo. In this letter, he claimed to be the only true Reiki teacher in Japan and accused specifically us, his teachers, of charlatanism. During the following year-and-a-half, just the mention of his name turned my eyes into balls of fire and caused my ears to smoke. It was the shock of my life: I had seen him as my friend, had energetically connected with him during his apprenticeship, the initiations, and exercises, felt him in my heart, and he slandered me in front of people whom neither he nor I knew. He wrote me a letter saying that while we practiced the initiations, he had looked at my hand and read the lines there. In my hand, he had seen how inferior I was in comparison to him and that my mind would not manage to understand him. It was the first time in my life as an adult that someone wanted to intentionally hurt me. I had spent so many years in Osho's ashram that something like this was completely foreign to me. That the attacker was also a student of Osho's was really the last straw. Today, three years later, I have to laugh heartily at the entire story. But back then I did not think it was funny at all. I felt myself injured in my soul and was disappointed at the ingratitude of humanity. Fortunately, life was kind enough to give me a number of valuable friends at that time, without whose love and affection I would certainly have withdrawn from my work as a Reiki teacher.

The result of this "negative" experience was that the mirror of self-contemplation was held in front of me, and I got to see my conditioning in a crystal-clear and distinct way. I had lived in an intact dream world of good knights and sweet fairies! I had practically gotten stuck in my heart chakra and no longer saw the entirety of life. I had been so imprinted by the strong Christianity morality of the good in contrast to the bad that I did not understand the harmony of yin and yang, sun and moon, and feminine and masculine. I believed that opposites excluded each other. Now I learned that opposites don't neutralize each other but mutually intensify and accentuate each other. Light does need darkness in order to exist.

I had put my friends on a pedestal throughout my life, idealized them, and was not willing to see their mistakes and weaknesses. Chetna often teased me about saying "but he/she is such a good person" when talking about a friend.

Even at an early age, I had a sunny character. The assistants in kindergarten said I was the happiest child they had met in their entire careers. On the other hand, being happy was also a trick that I had learned as a child to get the attention of adults and other children. I simply did not want to know about the negative aspects of life, let alone see them. In the final analysis, this experience gave me the opportunity of analyzing myself and reconsidering my rigid philosophy of life with its prefabricated moral attitude of good and evil. I learned to see other people with more clarity as they really are, without projecting my dreams on them.

At the end of September 1994, I flew to Tokyo to personally visit the grave of Dr. Usui in the cemetery of the Saihoji Temple and pay him my respects. Reiki had changed my life, and I simply wanted to thank him for this. Up to that day, my relationship to Dr. Usui had been an impersonal one that had always gone through a mediator. As I stood at Dr. Usui's grave with two Japanese friends and the light of Reiki permeated me, everything changed. After my excitement had settled down a bit, I rather naively asked my friends to translate the memorial stone on Usui's grave. Letters are letters, so I thought.

Unfortunately, this was not the case: even with their united powers, the two of them could only decipher a fraction of the epitaph since it was written in ancient Japanese. I was terribly disappointed because I have the tendency to always want everything right away. Luckily, I had brought my video camera and two other cameras along. I took detailed photos and film footage of the entire epitaph and had them developed the next day in Sapporo.

Chetna did not have much more luck in translating the epitaph than our friends, and so we asked her mother to translate the text, which is illustrated in my first book, Reiki Fire. I recently heard of a Dutch Reiki teacher (who speaks no Japanese!) claiming that we did not translate and print the entire text, but this absolutely is untrue. I just cannot understand how someone could pass on such an easily disprovable piece of nonsense.

The translation took a few weeks, and I became increasingly excited. Finally, there was something irrevocable from Dr. Usui, something in writing, as well as having been written in February 1927 by Dr. Usui's direct successor Ushida! I was spellbound. The memorial stone, which was placed there on the first anniversary of Dr. Usui's death by his organization and is still cared for by it today, has cleared away many of the Reiki tales. The doubts about Dr. Usui's legacy grew increasingly within me, but I had to still be patient for a while.

With time, I became increasingly sensitive about energy in general. One day, on the way to work, I suddenly felt a strong tingling pulsation in both hand chakras. I can still see myself today there in my car as I stared at my hands while waiting for the traffic light. I had the feeling that the palms of my hands were going to start burning at any moment. At first, I thought this phenomenon was physical energy that wanted to tell me something. However, when I got to the office and listened to our answering machine, a surprise awaited me: someone who wanted to learn Reiki had called precisely at the moment that I had experienced my tingling hands in the car. At first, I naturally considered this to be a coincidence. But when this occurrence repeated itself in the same way time and again, I become suspicious. Every time that my hands began to tingle, I listened to the answering machine at our school using the remote control—and each time someone had registered for Reiki. After a while, I lost interest in this game and no longer paid attention to it. Now my hand chakras are "active" throughout the entire day, even if there is nothing to do!

In the winter of 1994, I began to feel the energy flow in the meridians of my arms and legs. I asked my parents to send me a book about acupuncture and discovered that my experiences matched those of this ancient Chinese healing art. Feeling the energy currents is apparently mainly related to the attentiveness that a person gives his body and the subtle energy. However, in my opinion, energy phenomenon are not all that significant. They can help us better understand the human body and possibly let it receive energy when it has become unbalanced. The more sensitive a person is, the more beautiful and intensive every moment of life becomes. But we should not forget that the person who experiences the phenomenon is more important than the experience!

Some of the chakras that I had not felt at all or hardly felt earlier now made themselves noticeable. Above all, I felt the crown chakra during the Reiki initiations, my daily meditation, and whenever I used the master symbol.

I began to increasingly feel like an energy channel. With this feeling came a trace of modesty into my life. This energy apparently was not "mine" and this meant that there was no reason for the ego to want to distinguish itself as a result.

At this point, I would like to mention that it isn't important to notice or not notice a certain chakra. I often heard my master Osho say that we only feel certain energy centers when we are tense. In a relaxed channel, the energy flows unimpeded.

I have often heard from people interested in spirituality that the one chakra or the other is open or closed. But the matter isn't all that simple: It is said that every chakra in each of the seven bodies can be open or closed. This gives us 49 different possibilities!

Osho once responded to a student's question about the forehead chakra by saying that someone with a totally open forehead chakra is a saint. He lives beyond good and evil, has transcended sex, and is permanently immersed in ego-less divinity. Who can say that about himself—I certainly could not! For this person, dream and reality would be one and everything that she or he imagined would manifest itself immediately.

Most of my inner changes have taken place in an extremely peaceful manner and without any activity on my part. I often hardly noticed them until they had happened. The "aha" experiences came with increasing frequency. Reiki is such a gentle method of personal development and therefore completely safe and harmless for someone alone on the path. Other paths like yoga and certain methods of meditation should only be taken under the direction of a capable teacher or, even better, illuminated by the light of a spiritual master.

During the course of the years, I have become increasingly sensitive to the energy of people, animals, plants, places, things, and machines. Now when I pick up my car from an oil change, I always feel the intensified energy of the car. The more energy you put into a machine, a person, a relationship, a place, or a thing, the higher and more subtle the vibrations will become. And higher vibrations mutually attract each other. The German mystic Rudolf Steiner said somewhere that the thoughts we think often take on a life of their own as a result.

Sensitivity is not a spiritual, occult, or supernatural achievement but purely and simply the nature and birthright of every human being. The same applies to Reiki: it can be practiced by anyone, no matter who, where, or what he or she is.

In Japan, there is a wide-spread custom that prescribes giving gifts to business friends at Christmas and/or in the summer. Since we come into contact with quite a diversity of people because of our business, we receive a heap of presents twice a year. The energy attached to these things varies enormously. Things that have been selected and given with love are filled with love and light. Gifts that have been purchased from a sense of obligation feel like dead matter and need to be enriched with Reiki before using them.

The same approach should also be used for meals that have been cooked without love. In India, there is a custom that Brahmans should only eat food cooked by Brahmans. As I understand it, this is a bad "translation" of this old and wonderful custom. As has happened to the world religions, the true reason for enriching any type of nourishment—whether it is physical, emotional, or mental—with love has been lost during the course of the millennia. Only the outer form of this has remained, like the cast-off skin of a snake. Food that is prepared with love nourishes not only our physical body but also the divine within us.

When I go into a bookstore to look for literature on a particular topic, I first take each book in my hands and feel its energy. If it doesn't feel good to me, it gets put right back on the shelf.

Years ago, I already began tuning in to and conversing with our potted plants. The results can't be denied. Everyone who visits our school or home for the first time is enthused by the vitality of our plants. The house and office look more like a tropical garden. Maintaining this state has become even simpler through Reiki: Using the distance-healing symbol, connect with the plant, send it the mental-healing symbol, and seal it all with the power symbol. Now remain open and ask the plant how it's doing, if it likes the place where it's standing, whether it has enough sun and light, and so on. It may sound a bit far out to talk to the plants, but if you don't take it too seriously, it's just plain fun. It always brings me back to a state of carefree childhood, which I very much value.

If I find the time, during the warm summer months I like to sit under a certain tree in the park in front of our house before I go to sleep. Many trees have a wonderfully calming energy. The vitality that gently showers down on me from this tree is so overwhelming that tears of gratitude often run down my cheeks.

Not only living things can be charged with a clearly tangible energy capable of increasing or diminishing our well-being. As a child, I was very excited about prehistoric monuments. My parents showed my brother and me many Celtic cult and pilgrimage sites in Germany such as the Extern Stones in the vicinity of Detmold. Among other things, we also travelled to Stonehenge in England and Carnac in France. At that time, I didn't consciously feel the energy of these places. They appealed to my childlike sense of adventure and stimulated my fantasies. So I was joyfully surprised when we discovered some beautiful stone circles close to Sapporo several years ago. The Japanese are hardly interested in prehistoric culture, perhaps because it reminds them of a dark chapter in Hokkaido's history. The islands had been settled by the Ainu, a non-Japanese tribe that was practically exterminated in the most cruel manner within the past 200 years. Today, this fact is hushed up. These prehistoric cult sites are completely unknown and therefore frequently deserted. Whenever we feel particularly weary and drained, we get into the car and visit one of these mysterious power places in order to meditate there.

On several occasions, I have used the Second Degree (distance-healing symbol, the name of the place, mental-healing symbol, power symbol) to connect with the place and ask for advice. We've also carried out Reiki initiations there.

Through the years, I have learned to respect my body and listen to it. Our bodies have their own inherent wisdom, and it's worth getting in touch with this. As an experiment, use the distance-healing symbol to connect with the inner wisdom of your body, send it the mental-healing symbol as a gift, and seal the whole thing with the power symbol. Ask your body what you want to know and listen to it in silent reverence. At the beginning, it may not be easy to differentiate between the inner voice and imagination. I still have a hard time with this today. It's probably easier for women than for men, but intuition isn't reserved just for women. We all have it within us.

After you have talked to your body, thank it for the advice. As a rule, you should never connect with and talk to a disease since that would just give it more energy than it already claims for itself.

Before I learned Reiki, I ate excessive amounts of food. Although I have never been overweight in my life and have been a vegetarian since 1979, I didn't give much thought to the "what" and, above all, to the "how" of eating. We often went out to eat during the first years after we opened our school. This had always been something special to me ever since childhood, since I felt it to be identical with special holidays or vacations in foreign countries.

The more I came into contact with Reiki, the more difficult eating in restaurants became. I often felt bad after eating food that had been cooked without love. The energy just wasn't right. For the past three years, we either have been eating at home as much as possible or in restaurants where we personally know the cook.

The Third Step

More and more Reiki teachers, almost exclusively teachers who had been trained by us or our students, began offering their services in esoteric or New Age magazines. At that time, we had very consciously created our own "competition" because we didn't want to build up a sect-like organization with the two of us as gurus. Particularly in an area like Reiki, which involves peoples' religious feelings, I consider the formation of a rigid organization to be extremely dangerous and not at all in keeping with the purpose. When I noticed that I was no longer "the only" Reiki teacher in Japan, I suddenly felt insecure and depressed. I had to learn to let go of the position that I had created for myself. This wasn't a problem at all for Chetna... For me as a man with the wish and the will for power, it was an interesting time. Afterwards, we were doubly happy that we hadn't built up a Reiki organization at the time, even though this would certainly have been well-received in Japan. It's very easy to enthuse the Japanese for group dynamics and the related "disappearing in the crowd." Individuality isn't normally promoted. There is an old saying in Japan: "The nail that sticks out will get pounded in."

My best teachers were former students who maintained contact and shared their experiences with us after they had begun to teach on their own. I am sincerely thankful to them for this. Gradually, a wonderful Reiki network has been created with the Reiki teachers in all of Japan, America, Australia, Europe, Canada, and India.

Although we had decided to teach the Reiki Teacher Degree to anyone who wanted to learn it, the desire for control rose up inside of me when the first irresponsible Reiki teachers appeared on the scene. One of these teachers claimed in his advertising that people initiated into Reiki would probably never have to go to a doctor again for the rest of their lives. Others boasted that they could make cancer, AIDS, depressions, and other serious illnesses disappear with Reiki. This is naturally complete nonsense and shouldn't be taken seriously. Other Reiki teachers totally changed or completely dropped the initiations, which resulted in some of their students not experiencing the flow of energy and having to have a follow-up initiation.

In a conversation with my old friend and author Kirti Peter Michel, he recently explained to me his standpoint about the purpose of the initiations: they are mainly meant to guide our attention in a certain direction, the direction of spiritual awareness.

In his opinion, this concentrates the energy and brings it into a usable form. This is also an explanation for the diversity of rituals in the various Reiki schools. More than one way is possible: I myself have successfully tried out five different rituals. But a soundly tested and well-functioning ritual must be used! However, the most important aspect of the initiation is the teacher.

The Fourth Step

In August of 1995, our friend Shizuko Akimoto, who had learned Reiki from Chetna and with whom we work closely, met with Mr. Tsutomo Oishi, who had learned Reiki more than 30 years ago. Mr. Oishi had come to Shizuko, a wonderful healer, for a healing session. He suddenly began to speak about Reiki, without knowing that Shizuko is a Reiki teacher herself. Mr. Oishi introduced Shizuko to a Mr. Fumio Ogawa, whose adoptive father Kozo Ogawa had been a close colleague of Dr. Usui's and the chairman of the Reiki community in Shizuoka. As a result, more and more information came to light every week. With one forceful blow, the suspicion that had been gnawing at me since the "rediscovery" of Dr. Usui's grave the year before became certainty:

Mr. Chuyiro Hayashi had never been appointed as the successor to Usui! The actual successor had been Mr. Ushida. My Reiki world fell apart at this point. Although I had suspected it, I was still shocked: The teacher of my first Reiki teacher had also come from the Reiki Alliance, and now I had a problem! I felt deceived and illegitimate. I was afraid I had learned the "wrong" Reiki. After Shizuko had given Mr. Oishi a Reiki treatment that he very much liked, I became secure once again. Energetically, there simply isn't a difference between the one Reiki and the other.

It's clear to me that many Reiki teachers will be very critical toward this new information. I don't think that we should believe everything that we read or hear, as long as it can't be proved. A good portion of skepticism is certainly healthy. But in this case, the truth may be unpleasant for some of us, but this doesn't make it any less true. Not for a moment have I ever doubted that we all deserve hearing the truth and nothing but the truth. I know that I'm not the first person to examine the history of Reiki since Ms. Koyama and Mr. Ogawa have already been questioned regarding their knowledge before me (as early as 1985!) by other Western Reiki teachers or Reiki teachers who live in the West. I can't understand or accept why the truth hasn't been communicated to the Western Reiki world.

The Fifth Step

In Spring of 1996 I was deluged with letters, calls, and inquiries from German Reiki teachers who wanted to know more about the Japanese Reiki history.

The strangest letter came from a German Reiki teacher who wanted to legally protect (patent) the word "Reiki" and wrote me that he wouldn't accept me as a Reiki teacher if I couldn't prove my Reiki lineage back to Ms. Takata. I couldn't believe my eyes. The phrase "keeping Reiki clean" and the style of the letter reminded me of the Third Reich. I don't want to be a Reiki-Aryan!

Since I already knew that Mr. Chuyiro Hayashi and Ms. Takata who had followed him were not Reiki Grand Masters, Usui successors, or however we want to formulate it, I wasn't afraid of not being accepted as a Reiki teacher by someone in Germany. I only hoped that the whole talk about the true Reiki line and Reiki lines in general would finally stop.

I myself can trace back parts of my family for about eight hundred years. This brings me neither satisfaction, ability, happiness in life, nor more quality of life. Some of my ancestors were certain to have had an unpleasant nature. The same is the case with Reiki and our Reiki ancestors. A Reiki family tree doesn't mean much to me. The only important thing is the spirit of Reiki, the gratitude toward one's own teacher, and above all, the intensity with which we open ourselves up to the life energy in all of its aspects.

One day I received a call from Walter Lübeck, one of the most renowned German Reiki teachers and authors. My secretary asked him on the telephone to call back again since I was teaching at that moment. His response was: "No, I won't call back. I'm calling from Germany." As a good Japanese, my secretary was no match for this reply and put him through. I found his response to be quite good and laughed as I went to the telephone, which was a good start for us. We talked about Reiki in general for a while and then about my research here in Japan. I immediately felt connected with him. It was as if we already had known each other for a longer time and had just lost sight of each other for a while.

I had more or less finished writing my book The Reiki Fire in 1995, but hadn't been able to find a suitable publisher for it in Japan. Through a student, I had originally been asked to write a book about Reiki by a Japanese publisher since there were no Reiki books on the market at that time.

However, I was repulsed by the way in which the manuscript was treated by the publishing company. My words were twisted beyond recognition since they wanted my help in taking advantage of the booming Qigong trend in Japan. But I wasn't interested in doing this.

I broke off the relationship and immediately had another negative experience with a different publisher before I completely gave up. Walter now told me that the Windpferd Publishing in Germany was probably interested in a project with me. It hadn't been my intention to publish the book in Germany because I thought there were already enough Reiki books there. But that's how life goes sometimes.

Walter arranged a conversation with Windpferd, and within a few months I had signed a contact. At first, I was somewhat mistrusting, particularly since I had just read an American "how-to" book on publishing your own works. It urgently warned that authors are subject to deception everywhere. But this probably had more to do with the fear of the "how-to" book's author than reality.

A giant stone fell from my heart when I signed the contract. I had carried the book around inside of me for years, and now I was finally freed of it.

I immediately plunged into a new adventure and wrote, in addition to the poems that I have written since my childhood, a book about alternative education that hasn't yet been published. Its title is Be Yourself.

When we visited Germany in the summer of 1996, we also went to see Walter and his family in order to deepen our telephone friendship.

Without him, the Reiki Fire would never have become inflamed, and I wanted to personally thank him for this. We decided to continue working together, and then reluctantly went our separate ways. We had so much to discuss with each other!

In addition to Walter, we also met Wilfried M. Zapp, the musician who recorded and distributes the wonderful Reiki CD Oilios. This visit was just as warm and sincere, and I was happy that the three of us, who all had drawn from different sources of the Reiki family, could become friends. In our own way, we all work on more clarity and quality of life for ourselves personally and for others. It would be ridiculous if we couldn't do this together. During this year, the first non-Japanese came to us to learn Reiki. The network is slowly spanning the entire world.

The Reiki Fire was finally published by Windpferd in Germany in the middle of April 1997. The first very unpleasant reactions came within a week from functionaries of a large Reiki organization. But otherwise, the feedback that reached me was positive. Walter Lübeck had already warned me beforehand that the book would make some waves. He feared that the book would initially drive the Reiki fronts further apart before people could find their way back together. But reality is always more impressive than we can imagine: from America and Holland came accusations that I had violated "secret Japanese customs" (which don't even exist) and the publishing company was threatened with the courts if it didn't withdraw the book. I had "desecrated" Dr. Usui's grave with the publication, and so on and so forth. However, no one was hurt by my publication in Japan. After all, the memorial stone at Dr. Usui's grave was erected to inform the public about his life and work!

I was deeply shocked by these reactions since the reason for my research had been to finally bring to light the truth about Reiki history.

Now I had to understand that certain Reiki teachers were not at all interested in the actual truth but just wanted to protect their own interests. They had other things in mind and preferred to cling to the old Reiki tales. How else could this be possible?

Fortunately, many Reiki teachers sent me enthusiastic letters and thanked me for my work while just a few big Reiki fish wanted to go for my throat. I had apparently attacked power structures with the book, and these people were now desperately trying to defend them. Once again, I was ready to give up on Reiki and devote myself to other things, but in the meantime our research had been running at full speed and increasingly more information came to light.

The Sixth Step

At the end of 1997, I met a traditional Reiki teacher who had learned Reiki about 25 years ago from a Luizo Kobayashi. Like many other Japanese Reiki teachers, he didn't want to be involved in the Reiki power struggles in any way and therefore asked me not to mention his name.

I, on the other hand, had already had enough of the Reiki war that had openly broken out in the meantime. I wanted to put a quick end to it before Reiki was dragged through the dirt even more in the public eye. What was going on in the name of Reiki throughout the entire world no longer had anything to do with Reiki.

I had asked many of my Reiki friends to send me all their previously unanswered questions about Reiki so that I could get answers to them in Tokyo and satisfy more than just my own hunger for knowledge. As a result, I learned some things about traditional Japanese Reiki, which are explained in the section of "The Traditional Reiki Degrees." The teacher showed me methods that had been employed in Japan back then and are still used, and I also received an initiation. After we had talked about everything under the sun for hours, out of the blue he began to sing. I became completely intoxicated from it. I closed my eyes and let myself be flooded by the energy. One hour later, as I sat in the subway, I had the feeling that someone had chiseled open the top of my head and energy pulsated like crazy in my forehead. A new Reiki adventure had begun for me.

I first went to Poona, India, to the Osho Ashram, in order to get some distance from the world. As always, the arrival in Mumbai was shocking: it was August 15, 1997, the fiftieth anniversary of India's independence.

The taxi drivers were on strike and no one knew how to get one. The police just said, "it's no problem" and I should just keep walking straight ahead. Everyone I asked sent me straight ahead, the heat was overwhelming, and the air smelled like frankincense and feces.

I had already seen a lady in the airplane who somehow caught my eye. It turned out that she was also on her way to the Osho commune, and we decided to take a taxi to Poona together. Once in the taxi, it turned out that she had the first two Reiki degrees as well and we had a great deal to tell each other: her Reiki teacher was the teacher of my first teacher's teacher. The rain beat down mercilessly on the roof and against the windows of the taxi, and I was too excited to sleep despite the long journey.

I spent the larger part of my time in India meditating. After two weeks, I returned to Japan, where I met the well-known American Reiki teacher William Rand. I picked him up at the international airport in Tokyo, and we visited Dr. Usui's grave together with our friend Shizuko Akimoto the next day. The weather was quite bad and it was pouring. In the afternoon, we wanted to take the Tokaido express train to Kyoto. We had gotten behind schedule at Dr. Usui's grave and were in danger of missing our train. Shizuko, who was kind enough to bring us to the train station, became a bit nervous. From the time the subway got into the main train station in Tokyo, we had five minutes until our express train departed from a distant track.

Once we sat laughing in the train, we discovered that we both had used the same Reiki method to reach the train. We had used the distance-healing symbol and connected ourselves with the following situation: we both sat totally relaxed in our reserved seats in the express train. So we had run like crazy with all of our luggage through the endless corridors filled with crowds of people, up and down stairs, and reached our train at the last second.

One thing that I very much enjoyed in the conversations with William was the fact that he used the word Reiki as a verb. This works very well in English: "Let's Reiki it." Reiki actually has the qualities of a verb since it implies the flowing of energy, change, transformation, recovery, and healing on all levels. I also strongly felt that William works toward bringing closer together all the people who practice Reiki, and I would like to thank him sincerely once again for doing this. In a time where many artificial lines of borders are being created in the Reiki world, it's particularly important to come together and work together. I also hope that my books will ultimately contribute toward remembering what we have in common and learning to let go of trivial egocentricity.

The next day, we met two additional friends, Laura Gifford and Friedemann Greulich, a friend of Laura's who oddly enough lives in my neighborhood.

We exchanged experiences and initiations on Kurama Mountain, at the place where the Kurama god Maoson supposedly came to Earth six million years ago. Whether it was because of the deity or the divinity in general—this was a great place.

It's possible to forget time here and, even though the temple facilities are quite overrun, no one bothers you.

During my first visit on the Kurama, I had been misled by my high expectations. Although I wasn't conscious of it at the time, I had probably expected a mystical experience on the Kurama and couldn't experience things as they actually were. It was completely different this time. The wonderful atmosphere was joined by splendid weather, the wonderful smell of the giant cedars mixed with incense sticks and the awareness of being completely protected, resting in the cradle of Reiki like a baby.

Once I was back again in Sapporo, which is located about 1,500 kilometers to the north of Kyoto, I found a half ton of mail waiting for me. The Reiki Fire had slowly caught on in the USA. Since we had included our address in the book, I was suddenly inundated with letters, faxes, and email. But the next big surprise was already in store. During the summer, Shizuko Akimoto had given us an old manuscript by Dr. Usui with the title of Usui Reiki Ryoho (see translation), which she had received from Mr. Oishi. Since I couldn't read it, Chetna had translated it during my absence. Reiki wasn't just an oral tradition—there was finally something from Dr. Usui personally!

This manuscript exceeded my expectations by far and I decided to write a second book about Reiki. I had actually been writing a novel, which I very much enjoyed. But now it was clear that this news wanted to be shared with all of you!

The Seventh Step
I spent the autumn of 1997 answering correspondence. The book had created quite a sensation, and I heard a great deal about us and our research from people who neither knew us nor were informed about our investigations and sources.

An American Reiki teacher claimed that we had received our information from a splinter group—I asked myself who this splinter group is, looking at the Reiki family tree

A Canadian Reiki teacher claimed that the picture in The Reiki Fire was a digital composition created in a computer, that Dr. Usui's memorial stone had only been installed during the Eighties and one of my first students, Toshitaka Mochizuki (who had done a great deal of research himself and had also written a book about Reiki with the title Iyashi No Te), was amused about the stupidity of my book.

Toshitaka, who had written me shortly before to say how good he found the book to be, was appalled to hear this and happy that he had already broken off contact with the Canadian a year before.

This time, I couldn't take the attacks seriously and remembered a Chinese classic in which false reports are suggested to be a very successful means of strategy. However, these false reports shouldn't be signed by the person circulating them ...

At the end of December 1997, I returned to Germany once again. I wanted to see my parents, the people at the publishing company, and some Reiki teachers and friends. For several weeks, I had been in quite an emotional state after seeing a picture of the Indian saint Ma Anandamayi Ma, which had intensely shaken me. I cried a great deal without any reason. It was simply like a full vessel overflowing, a rain cloud that emptied itself on a mountain slope, or a river that poured into the sea.

At this point, I would like to quote a few words from this saint, who unfortunately is quite unknown in the West:

"A saint is like a tree. He calls no one to himself, nor does he send anyone away. He offers to protect everyone who wants to come to him, whether this be a man, a woman, a child, or an animal. When you sit under a tree, it will protect you from the harshness of the weather, from both the heat of the sun and the pouring rain, and it will give you flowers and fruit.

Whether a human being is pleased at the sight of it or a bird eats from it is unimportant for the tree. Its gifts are there for everyone who comes and takes them. And it ultimately gives itself. How does this happen? The fruit contains seeds for a new tree of the same type. So you will, when you sit under a tree, receive protection, shade, flowers, and fruit, and you will recognize your own self at the appropriate time."

I can't foresee where my path in life may still lead me, and quite honestly, this makes no difference at all to me. I remember something written by Osho's hand, with which I want to close this chapter: "The journey itself is the goal."

Exercises

In the following chapter, I will describe some exercises that I consider helpful. They actually have nothing to do with Reiki, but they have been valuable help for me and other Reiki friends.

Exercise 1
Sit down in a quiet place and ask yourself: Who am I? Now try to answer this question within the course of half an hour. You will probably first say your own name and wonder how it is related to you. If it were to be removed from your consciousness, you would still be yourself so let go of it for the sake of the exercise. Now let your imagination run free. It will suggest an apparently endless amount of identification solutions; however, after clear reflection these repeatedly will turn out to be incorrect. You are neither your name, your body, your emotions, your memory, your dreams and desires, nor your possessions, your friends, your thoughts, or your future. All this ultimately turns out to be inadequate and you remain what you actually are: pure consciousness without names, attributes, valuations, and gender. You are free!

Exercise 2
Take a piece of paper and list on it everything that you have ever heard about the magical power of Reiki, but what you haven't experienced yourself. Now try to become clear about what you have assumed to be a given without ever questioning it. I don't want to stir up your mistrust here but encourage you to take your own path. Skepticism and mistrust are not always identical. A healthy pinch of skepticism makes life easier if you are simultaneously open for all the possibilities that life has to offer.

Almost every day, I also separate myself from the prejudices and knowledge of other people that I had taken on as my own truth. A thorough Reiki house-cleaning would probably be good for many of us.

Exercise 3
Think about what you want to change in your life and what you don't like about your life. Now ask yourself why this doesn't

appeal to you and what you would like to have instead of it. If a reason seems plausible to you, accept it and thank your subconscious mind for it. Now imagine how it would be if the undesired was separated from what you desire. Then take a piece of paper and simply start writing on it how this situation could be changed. Don't think that this thing or the other could be unrealistic and disregard your rational judgment for the time being.

When nothing more occurs to you, look at the list and choose the strategy for transformation that best appeals to you. Follow this path uncompromisingly for at least three months.

Exercise 4

Imagine that you are as open and uninhibited as a child. Try to remember your childhood or how you felt as a child. If you still have photos from your childhood, these may help you. Look at one of the pictures and attempt to remember the situation in which it was taken. Put yourself into this situation again and feel how you felt as a child. If you still have toys around from your childhood, use them for the same purpose. A teddy bear can often help you in a wonderful way as well.

As soon as you have a strong memory of the feeling of being a child, select a day in which you are surrounded only by your partner or a close friend and open your heart. Don't hold your feelings back. Cry, if you feel like it. And laugh when you feel like laughing. I don't recommend that you do this exercise while you are at work since you will probably be quite vulnerable and your colleagues may be offended by your emotions!

Exercise 5—Energy Exercises

If you think that you aren't sensitive enough to feel energy, don't worry. The sensing of the energy flow is like a muscle that each of us can train if we only want to. We don't need to first be a person who is "magnificently" developed when it comes to spirituality. Each of us can grasp energy at this moment with a little bit of practice.

Here is the exercise: Hold both of your hands away from your upper body with the palms facing each other at a distance of about one meter (yard). Do you feel something? If so, register it without getting lost in the feeling. If not, don't let yourself be confused by this. Let the energy flow between your hands for a few minutes. Now slowly let the palms come closer to each other and stop as soon as you feel a change. If not, hold them at a distance of fifty centimeters (one-and-a-half feet) for a few minutes. Feel the flow of energy. Now let the palms move a bit closer to each other again, this time to about twenty centimeters. Each time when you feel a change, stop your hands and become aware of the sensation. Finally, let the palms move even closer together and hold them at a distance of 3—5 centimeters (several inches) from each other. Now you will probably not only feel the "tingling," the vibrations of the energy, but also the warmth. If you feel nothing at all, then don't worry about it and practice again on another day.

According to my experience, even the initiation into the First Reiki Degree makes a big difference in the flow of energy for someone who hasn't been initiated into Reiki. The above exercise can also be done very well by two people.

In case you have completed the Second or Third Reiki Degree, you can also let the various Reiki symbols flow from your hands.

After you have clearly felt the energy between your hands, go one step further and hold one of your hands above a part of your body. Now proceed as described above.

Exercise 6
Greet everything and everyone as your teacher. There is nothing in life from which we can't learn. Whether health, disease, nature, human being, or animal—everyone and everything can become our teacher when we are open and willing to learn from life and all the possible (and sometimes impossible) situations.

Exercise 7
Under the shower: Wash not only the dust from your body but also from your soul. Imagine how the water takes all your worries and negative thoughts and feelings down the drain with it. While you stand under the shower and soap yourself, touch your body lovingly. There's no reason not to love your own body, the house of your soul! If you have learned the Second or Third Reiki Degree, project the mental-healing symbol or the master symbol into the spray of water and let yourself be charged by the energy.

Exercise 8

Osho said at some point that many traditional masters and spiritual paths demand of their students that they separate from their friends. Abstinence from sex, alcohol, cigarettes, coffee, and tea are wide-spread methods for directing the student's energy inwardly. However, according to Osho there is also another possibility: he simply asks us to let go of our suffering! This may sound tempting, but it isn't all that simple. Based on my own experience, I know how we desperately cling to what makes us sick and depressed, as crazy as this may seem, and stops us from becoming part of the light.

Exercise 9

The therapeutic effects of laughing, crying, and meditating have been thoroughly researched throughout the world in recent years. Psychotherapists in the East and West know that someone who lives in a balanced, relaxed, and meditative manner is physically healthier and maintains more harmonious relationships with his fellow human beings on the one hand, but also is more creative and works more effectively on the other hand.

When I went to Osho's ashram in India during the spring of 1988, he had developed a new meditation, the "Mystic Rose Meditation," meant to combine therapy and meditation. It consists of three parts, each of which lasts one week. In the first week, the participants were to laugh for three hours a day without any reason to do so. At least during the first five days, this part was quite easy for me. I will never forget the picture of about seventy adults rolling on the floor with laughter!

In the second week, the participants were to cry without any reason. At first, I had difficulty doing this. I hadn't cried publicly and without holding back since earliest childhood.

In the third week, we meditated with closed eyes while observing our breathing for three hours a day. After the two previous weeks with their daily emotional outbursts, the silence was unbelievably deep.

The results of this method are amazing, and I can most warmly recommend it to anyone interested in spiritual growth. Almost everyone with whom I discussed this method said that his life had changed fundamentally as a result.

Unfortunately, this meditation can't be performed alone. It should be done with a qualified therapist and, if at all possible,

in the seclusion of a therapy center or ashram. For further information, please contact the Osho Multiversity, Osho Commune International, 17 Koregaon Park, 411001 Poona Ms. India.
Fax: 91-212-624181
Email: cc.osho#oci.sprintrpg.ems.vsnl.net.in

Afterword

Now that we have finally found our Reiki roots, it's time for us to reach our arms toward the light together.

As lone fighters, it's much harder to progress on our inner journey. Growth takes place not only on an individual basis, but also on a collective basis. We can see this very clearly in a close relationship or a circle of spiritual seekers. A more intensive speed of growth is possible within a group that has the same spiritual objective, namely pursuing the goal of self-realization.

I'm not suggesting founding a new Reiki sect here, but that we stop making life difficult for each other, stop fighting each other, stop being unaccepting of each other and just seeing our "own" Reiki as the one true form.

The differences between the various Reiki currents shouldn't lead us to something like a holy war but to a celebration of the expanded possibilities of our collective consciousness.

As a group, we are capable of taking giant steps of development when we begin to primarily experience the spirit that lives within all of us and leave the triviality of discord behind.

I am certain that a great portion of humanity is mature enough to harmoniously dance into the twenty-first century. From my heart and soul, I wish all of you, dear dance partners, that the Existence continues to shower you with all its gifts, its love, and its light.

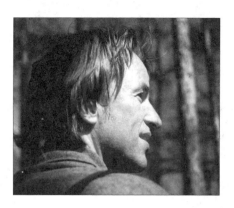

About the Author

Whether as an agricultural adviser in the hills of Oregon, a landscape gardener for Bill Gates in Washington, or a computer expert in New York, whether as a photographer or poet, Frank Arjava Petter, who has been a student of the Indian meditation master Osho since 1979, strives to perceive, shape, and heal inner qualities in the outer world.

At the beginning of 1993, he brought Reiki back to the land of its origin and started teaching the Reiki Master/Teacher Degree for the first time in Japan.

He currently lives with his Japanese wife in Sapporo, Northern Japan, where he heads an alternative language school and teaches various healing therapies and methods of meditation.

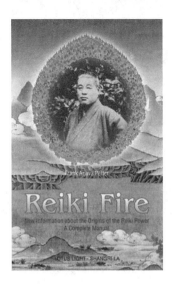

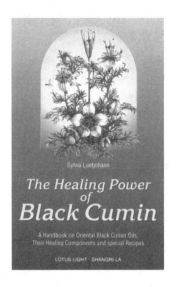

Frank Arjava Petter

Reiki Fire

**New Information about
the Origins of the Reiki Power
A Complete Manual**

The origin of Reiki has com to be surrounded by many stories and myths. The author, an independent Reiki Master practicing in Japan, immerses it in a new light as he traces Usui-san's path back through time with openness and devotion. He meets Usui's descendants and climbs the holy mountain of his enlightenment. Reiki, shaped by Shintoism, is a Buddhist expression of Qigong whereby Qigong depicts the teaching of life energy in its original sense. An excellent textbook, fresh and rousing in its spiritual perspective, this is an absolutely practical Reiki guide. The heart, the body, the mind, and esoteric background, are all covered here.

**144 pages - $12.95
ISBN: 978-0-9149-5550-4**

Walter Lübeck

The Healing Power
of Black Cumin

**A Handbook on Oriental Black
Cumin Oils, Their Healing
Components, and Special Recipes**

Long confirmed by good experiences, the sensational effects of black cumin (known also as black seed) oils have also been substantiated by modern science. Black cumin is an excellent healer. Its areas of application extend from skin care to the treatment of diseases of the skin and respiratory tract. In this comprehensive book, the most important types of black cumin oils are described with their specific effects through the use of many practical examples. Time-tested recipes for health and beauty care from both traditional and modern naturopathy, as well as many practical tips from black cumin experts, round off this valuable guide.

**176 pages - $14.95
ISBN: 978-0-9149-5553-5**

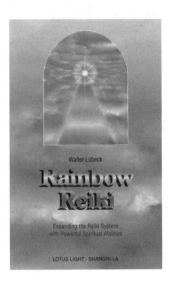

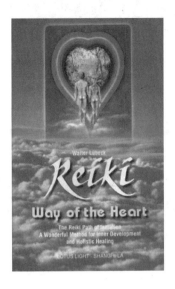

Walter Lübeck

Rainbow Reiki
Expanding the Reiki System
with Powerful Spiritual Abilities

Rainbow Reiki gives us a wealth of possibilities to achieve completely new and different things with Reiki than taught in the traditional system. Walter Lübeck has tested these new methods in practical application for years and teaches them in his courses. Making Reiki Essences, performing guided aura and chakra work, connecting with existing power places and creating new personal ones, as well as developing Reiki Mandalas, are all a part of this system. This work is accompanied by plants devas, crystal teachers, angels of healing stones, and other beings of the spiritual world.

192 pages - $14.95
ISBN: 978-0-9149-5528-3

Walter Lübeck

Reiki—Way of the Heart
The Reiki Path of Initiation
A Wonderful Method for Inner
Development and Holistic Healing

Reiki—Way of the Heart is for everyone interested in the opportunities and experiences offered by this very popular esoteric path of perception, based on easily learned exercises conveyed by a Reiki Master to students in three degrees.
If you practice Reiki, the use of universal life energy to heal oneself and others, you will have the possibility of receiving direct knowledge about your personal development, health, and transformation.
Walter Lübeck also presents a good survey of various Reiki schools and shows how Reiki can be applied successfully in many areas of life.

192 pages - $14.95
ISBN: 978-0-9145-2491-9

Music for Reiki Treatments

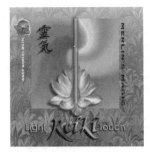

Reiki: Light Touch
Merlin's Magic

One of the most recommended music for Reiki treatments. This beautiful, serenely blissful instrumental music is a real gift for healing and happiness. It's soothing sounds and caressing vibratio:s are wonderful for so many forms of body work, energy balancing, meditation or even relaxing. Combining guitar, keyboards, violin, viola and deeply resonant Tibetan bells to create the relaxing sounds of LIGHT TOUCH.
60 min. Inner Worlds Music
MC ISBN: 978-0-9102-6179-1
CD ISBN: 978-0-9102-6185-2

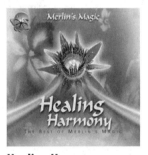

Healing Harmony
The Best of Merlin's Magic

Merlin's Magic is a proven best-seller. Now Merlin's Magic presents a wonderful follow-up compilation album to their best-selling former albums Reiki, Reiki Light Touch, Heart of Reiki and Angel Helpers. Also it presents two new compositions. This recording will delight you!
73 min. Inner Worlds Music
MC ISBN: 978-0-9102-6148-7
CD ISBN: 978-0-9102-6150-0

Reiki
Merlin's Magic

Reiki Music was specially composed and arranged to be played during Reiki treatments. However, because of its gentle, suggestive powers, it is an equally ideal background for other forms of bodywork and techniques of energy balancing.
60 min. Inner Worlds Music
MC ISBN: 978-0-9102-6181-4
CD ISBN: 978-0-9102-6187-6

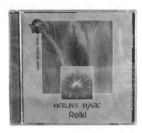

The Heart of Reiki
Merlin's Magic

The Heart of Reiki comes from the deepest centers of energy to touch the hearts of listeners and create the perfect balance of body, mind and soul. It's a powerful celebration of the ethereal Reiki energy, more healing and more blissful than ever.
One long session of music that is sure to relax and calm while invigorating. Perfect accompaniment for Reiki treatment of body work sessions of any kind.
60 min. Inner Worlds Music
MC ISBN: 978-0-9102-6153-1
CD ISBN: 978-0-9102-6152-4

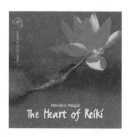

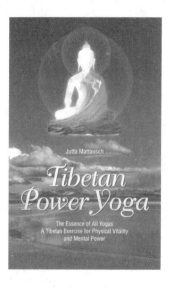

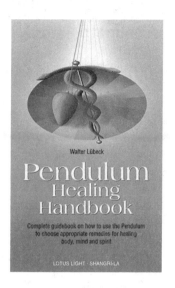

Jutta Mattausch

Tibetan Power Yoga

The Essence of All Yogas
A Tibetan Exercise for
Physical Vitality
and Mental Power

Here is an absorbing story set in distant
Tibet, and yet could also take place
within all of us anywhere in the world,
since it deals with the journey to the
self. Whether you arrive at yourself and
then perhaps also find yourself, depends on your willingness to open up...
This completely undogmatic book deals
with one of the oldest exercises in the
world, an exercise that is simple and
unique. "Tibetan Power Yoga" is what
the Tibetan Lama Tsering Norbu calls
this set of strong motions, similar to a
"great wave" that has given the people
from the Roof of the World physical vitality and mental power up into ripe old
age since time immemorial.

112 pages - $9.95
ISBN: 978-0-9149-5530-6

Walter Lübeck

Pendulum Healing Handbook

Complete guidebook on how to use
the Pendulum to choose appropriate
remedies for healing body, mind and
spirit

If you want to learn every aspect of how
to use a pendulum, particularly in relation to methods of alterative healing,
this book is for you.
This book contains many of the most
important pendulum tables from the areas of nutrition, aromas, Bach Flowers,
gemstones, chakras, herbs, relationships, etc., and shows how to use them,
along with the limits of their application.
Walter Lübeck begins with the selection
of the right pendulum, shows the correct way to hold it, and also explains
the possibilities of energetic cleansing.
With 125 pendulum tables.

208 pages - $15.95
ISBN: 978-0-9149-5554-2